EVERY STORY COUNTS

Exploring Contemporary Practice
Through Narrative Medicine

∞

Arthur Lazarus, MD, MBA, CPE

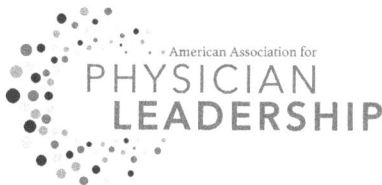

American Association for
PHYSICIAN
LEADERSHIP

PUBLISHER
Nancy Collins

PRODUCTION MANAGER
Jennifer Weiss

DESIGN & LAYOUT
Carter Publishing Studio

COPYEDITOR
Pat George

*In a life recounted by stories, this book
is dedicated with love to my children and
grandchildren, whose stories are still unfolding.*

*And to Cheryl, for bearing witness to
my stories since medical school.*

TABLE OF CONTENTS

EDUCATION AND TRAINING

HEALTH POLICY

PRACTICE MANAGEMENT

About the Author

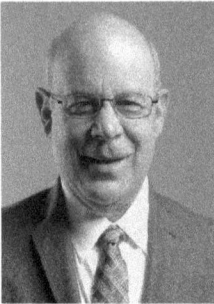

Arthur L. Lazarus, MD, MBA, CPE, DFAAPL, DLFAPA, is a healthcare consultant, certified physician executive, and nationally recognized author, speaker, and champion of physician leadership and wellness. He has broad experience in clinical practice and the health insurance industry, having led programs at Cigna and Humana. At Humana, Lazarus was vice president and corporate medical director of behavioral health operations in Louisville, Kentucky, and subsequently a population health medical director for the state of Florida.

Lazarus has also held leadership positions in several pharmaceutical companies, including Pfizer and AstraZeneca, conducting clinical trials, and reviewing promotional material for medical accuracy and FDA compliance. He has published more than 250 articles in scientific and professional journals and has written four books, including *Neuroleptic Malignant Syndrome and Related Conditions, Controversies in Managed Mental Health Care, Career Pathways in Psychiatry, and MD/MBA: Physicians on the New Frontier of Medical Management.*

Born in Philadelphia, Pennsylvania, Lazarus attended Boston University, where he graduated with a bachelor's degree in psychology with Distinction. He received his medical degree with Honors from Temple University School of Medicine, followed by a psychiatric residency at Temple University Hospital, where he was chief resident. After residency, Lazarus joined the faculty of Temple University School of Medicine, where he currently serves as adjunct professor of Psychiatry. He also holds non-faculty appointments as Executive-in-Residence at Temple University Fox School of Business and Management, where he received his MBA degree, and Senior Fellow, Jefferson College of Population Health, Philadelphia, Pennsylvania.

Well known for his leadership and medical management skills, Lazarus is a sought-after presenter, mentor, teacher, and writer. He has shared his expertise and perspective at numerous local, national, and international meetings and seminars.

Lazarus is a past president of the American Association for Psychiatric Administration and Leadership, a former member of the board of directors of the American Association for Physician Leadership (AAPL), and a current member of the AAPL editorial review board. In 2010, the American Psychiatric Association honored Lazarus with the Administrative Psychiatry Award for his effectiveness as an administrator of major mental health programs and expanding the body of knowledge of management science in mental health services delivery systems.

Lazarus is among a select group of physicians in the United States who have been inducted into both the Alpha Omega Alpha medical honor society and the Beta Gamma Sigma honor society of collegiate schools of business.

Lazarus lives with his wife near Charlotte, North Carolina. They have four adult children. He enjoys walking, biking, playing piano, and listening to music.

Contact Dr. Lazarus at artlazarus6@gmail.com.

Acknowledgments

I am grateful to Kevin Pho, MD, founder of KevinMD, for amplifying my voice by allowing me to share my insight and tell my stories to his loyal community of readers: physicians, advanced practitioners, nurses, medical students, and patients.

At MedPage Today, Genevieve Friedman has been an invaluable editor and adviser. Thanks, Jenny, for sharpening my viewpoints, elevating my perspectives, and placing missing commas.

To the editorial team at Doximity, thanks for your trust and confidence in my writing and for delivering on your mission to put the "clinician first."

Peter Angood, MD, president and chief executive officer of the American Association for Physician Leadership, and Nancy Collins, senior vice president of content development and acquisition, have been good friends for over a decade. Their ongoing support and encouragement were instrumental in the publication of this book.

FOREWORD

By Peter B. Angood, MD

THERE IS NO DOUBT HEALTHCARE is the most complex of industries — one that continues to grapple with longstanding and emerging challenges that, in many cases, require physicians' viewpoints to help find effective solutions. In this often-perplexing environment, the unique expertise and perspective of physician leadership provide added value and benefits well-proven during the past few decades.

Physician leadership is more important than ever.

I believe that all physicians are leaders at some level. Physicians and the patient–physician relationship are the dominant drivers of today's healthcare industry. Physicians have dedicated their lives to helping others, and they are ready and willing to help their practices and organizations continue to meet the challenges of the day.

Regardless of clinical commitment, administrative responsibilities, or professional level (in both titled and non-titled roles), who better to provide expanded leadership and stewardship of this industry than the physicians who are its natural and historical leaders?

Each of us, in our own way, has been sharing in this leadership (perhaps unknowingly) by utilizing storytelling to gain or provide clinical and administrative insights throughout our careers. This leadership sharing is typically through the stories we call interesting cases or case studies.

There has been a circle of successful physician storytellers/writers throughout time: W. Somerset Maugham, Anton Chekhov, poets John Keats and William Carlos Williams, and Sir Arthur Conan Doyle, who created Sherlock Holmes and his physician sidekick, Dr. Watson. More contemporary physician storytellers include Richard Selzer, Sherwin B. Nuland, Oliver Sacks, Atul Gawande, Abraham Verghese, Khaled Hosseini, Robin Cook, Perri Klass, Danielle Ofri, Rita Charon, Rachel Naomi Remen, and the late Michael Crichton.

With his rich background of professional and personal experiences as a physician and medical leader, Art Lazarus has developed his own storytelling style and now shares his perceptions with this book, *Every Story Counts*. The book is a collection of essays that provide insights and commentary across several elements of healthcare that will resonate on some level with most physicians, young and old. For young physicians, it's like having a sage advisor in your pocket; for those further along, it's akin to having a wise peer assure us that we are not alone, as each of us has experienced similar influences and reacted accordingly. And we can each be challenged occasionally by these discerning reflections and questions posed.

This collection of 76 essays is organized into six focus areas:
1. Physician Issues
2. Professional Development
3. Education and Training
4. Health Policy
5. Patient Care
6. Practice Management

Individually and collectively, the essays across these focus areas provide a unique viewpoint of our industry and the variety of issues that each of us should pay attention to during our career trajectories. The breadth of issues is covered succinctly and with enough depth to make the entire book a worthwhile read for those in medicine, as well as for those wishing to learn more about physicians in this industry.

Narrative medicine has evolved rapidly as a nuanced, but intriguing utilization of storytelling. Clinicians from a variety of disciplines have found the art of narrative medicine to be not only a channel for creativity but also a form of therapy when dealing with the many tribulations of modern medicine. Dr. Lazarus's collection of essays provides a complexion of both — they are creative and thought-provoking, yet simultaneously soothing and calming.

The medical profession is viewed as a leadership profession not only by our industry, but also by general society. Therefore, as physician leaders, we must embrace the complexities of our industry. And we can choose to embrace the opportunities in which our energies are able to create the positive transformation needed for our industry.

Sharing our stories and experiences is an essential component of the physician leadership fabric. Dr. Lazarus provides a delightfully bright thread to help each of us hold the fabric together over time. Physicians, their families, and their patients will all benefit — directly or indirectly — from reading this book.

PREFACE

IN MAY 2019, ABOUT SIX MONTHS before COVID-19 struck, I was stricken by my own crisis, certainly nowhere near the magnitude of a global pandemic, but a personal setback, nevertheless. I lost my job at an insurance company. It wasn't the first time my position had been eliminated, but unlike previous instances, I was totally unprepared and caught off-guard. I knew the company was losing money and downsizing, and there were rumors of a buyout, but I went about my business working remotely from home, shielded from the scuttlebutt. Then the phone call came informing me of the bad news.

I was unemployed for nearly a year. The job I eventually landed was one I invented to save face: an independent consultant — not exactly the prestigious title I had been accustomed to in academic practice and the corporate world. I figured ageism was to blame for my difficulty in finding full-time employment because, after all, I qualify for Medicare and collect Social Security income. Besides, my age can easily be interpolated from dates listed on employment applications, e.g., graduation from college, medical school, and residency. I felt stonewalled from re-entering the work force. It became such a significant source of frustration that I began to write to sooth my soul. I was very mindful of what Maya Angelou had to say about bearing an untold story: "There is no greater agony."

Unemployment and age discrimination are two of many topics I began to explore using narrative medicine as a tool to communicate challenges most physicians confront at some point in their career. Depicting scenarios that are evergreen — ones that resonate with generations of physicians even as medical knowledge expands and is updated — was foremost on my mind. Although the generation gap is real and widening, the foundation of medicine and what it means to be a doctor has hardly changed since Hippocrates' time. (In "Precepts," Hippocrates declared: "…where there is love of man, there is also love of the art. For some patients, though conscious that their condition is perilous, recover their health simply through their contentment with the goodness of the physician.")

Another goal in writing was to use storytelling to contextualize important themes in medical education, training, and practice, as well as health policy and practice management. I thought it was relevant to address both clinical and nonclinical aspects of practice and to refer to key findings and observations, where appropriate, to support my views. Examining the inner-workings of contemporary practice and the transformation wrought by the "medical-industrial complex" proved to be enlightening, if not disheartening. As you will see, many physicians perceive the U.S. medical system to be broken and flawed, built on exploiting the values that brought them into the field in the first place.

Certainly, the events I witnessed prior to and since that fateful call in 2019 — indeed, the collective experience of physicians during the coronavirus pandemic — remind us that every story counts. But, as J. K. Rowling points out, "No story lives unless someone wants to listen." So, I offer you stories of impact, from the time physicians prepare for a life's calling until they retire, stories in which they see parts of themselves and others close to them. I hope the essays in this book compel you to think about your present and future career, and along with it, the inevitable satisfaction of a successful journey.

Physician Issues

∞

I Am Not What Others Think of Me

The idea of proving others wrong motivates many of us, but it's unhealthy. Besides, continuously proving that people have underestimated your abilities is exhausting. Learn early how to cast away self-doubt and believe in yourself.

I ALWAYS HAD AN EYE toward medical school, even though I majored in psychology in college. I didn't have the fortitude for rigorous science courses, and I preferred to party on campus rather than study. After all, this was the early 1970s. Entering my junior year with an overall 3.4 GPA (lower for the science courses), I was told by my pre-med adviser that I'd never get into medical school. It hadn't occurred to me until then that she may be right. I buckled down, but not in time to reverse the damage of two years of mediocre scholastic performance. All medical schools rejected me.

My adviser's comment stuck in my head, and I was determined to prove her wrong. I spent a year taking additional science courses, studying to retake the MCATs, and working part-time at a Harvard-affiliated hospital. I figured it couldn't hurt to have a recommendation or two written on Harvard University letterhead.

The combination of hard work and determination paved my way into medical school. Compared to many of my peers of that era who either went to medical school abroad and languished for several years before they were accepted into a U.S. school or abandoned their dreams of becoming a doctor, I suppose I was fortunate.

The need to prove people wrong became a source of motivation for me. It helped me excel in medical school, residency, and beyond. By continually displaying my skills, I was able to disprove my critics. However, trying to prove people wrong all the time was exhausting, and it spurred me into academic and professional competitions so intense that I lost friendships and relationships.

I can say I truly wanted to become a doctor, which was not the case for other clinicians. Some were motivated to attend medical school simply because others told them they couldn't cut it, a family member looked down on them because they didn't want to follow tradition, or maybe they wanted to become a nurse.

Think about it: In the excitement of proving people wrong, acting out of revenge becomes a total waste of time and resources if you become a doctor without having a genuine interest in medicine. You will regret your career choice and may not treat your patients well. Here is yet another reason for someone to prove you wrong and demoralize you. Nevertheless, seeking revenge on doubters and non-believers is constantly played up in the media and in songs and movies.

Where does the desire to prove people wrong originate? Most experts agree it's during the school years: experiences with difficult teachers and interactions with peers who tease and taunt, as I describe in essay 26. I endured hurtful name-calling in high school due to my weight. It's no wonder the dour outlook proffered by my pre-med adviser rekindled painful memories and shaped a future in which I felt destined to prove everyone wrong. My professor's pronouncement was my main drive to succeed, and it worked.

The important question, however, is whether the end justifies the means. Is proving other people wrong healthy or harmful to your psyche? My training in psychiatry suggests you shouldn't get your energy from negative people because it's easier to use other people's negativity as fuel than it is to search within yourself and hone your native abilities. It's more difficult to overcome feelings of insecurity and build confidence from a foundation of strength than it is to want people to like you for what you've achieved.

Over time, I gained confidence by writing and publishing books and articles, speaking at professional organizations, and being elected to leadership roles in medical societies. I rose to the rank of professor. As I became surer of my talents, abilities, and accomplishments, other people's opinions didn't matter that much to me, and the need to prove them wrong dissipated.

I'd like to think I've paid it forward to students and residents by mentoring them and furthering their self-actualization, thus sparing them the distress I suffered early in my career. I advise them that if they simply exist to negate others' opinions, it serves as a vital clue that they probably have some work to do in terms of valuing their self-worth.

Chances are, there is (or was) a lingering negative force in your life. It may be human nature to want to prove people wrong, but making someone else wrong doesn't necessarily make you right. Perhaps the greatest motivator of all is to succeed for yourself on your own terms. Prove to yourself — not to others — that people are wrong about you and, in the process, help them find their own motivation to change.

Some Doctors Need Lessons in Civility

The internet can be a safe haven for your writing, but it can also be a place where you are viciously attacked for your views. Follow the golden rule when responding to someone's remarks: "Do unto others as you would have them do unto you."

WHEN I LEFT TRADITIONAL EMPLOYMENT, I discovered I didn't have to answer to anyone other than myself and my family. I felt a certain freedom to speak up more than ever. I was mostly concerned with the ill health of physicians — not "wellness," because many physicians are actually unwell — and how practicing has exacted a terrible toll on the emotional health of physicians manifesting in burnout, depression, suicide, PTSD, and substance use.

Because I had more time on my hands. I began visiting several medical blogs on a regular basis. I soon detected another malady that afflicts doctors, and it's not pretty. It has to do with the way physicians attack each other on online social media platforms. Physicians, it seems, are just not civil to one another in many instances.

An essay I wrote for Doximity, published August 7, 2021 (essay 62 in this book), resonated with many doctors. One physician responded, "You have written in that article everything that we all who suffer the same conditions [fearing to speak out] would want to write. THANKS SO MUCH FOR BEING OUR VOICE."

Another physician sent me a private message, saying, "I just read your article about speaking out. Thank you. It came at a really good time for me. I've learned a lot about censorship recently and trying to figure out how to proceed." Make no mistake about it. Doctors have been harshly censored, especially for speaking out about how their employers mishandled the initial phases of COVID-19 preparedness.

However, a few doctors took issue with my essay and had some really nasty things to say. One said, "I find it hard to believe that you can work for 40 years and 'not speak up' and feel that it is ok...I wonder how many patients were harmed by not speaking up for 40 years." Another physician critiqued my essay for being "internally inconsistent" and suggested my motivation for writing it was less than altruistic. We argued back and forth online until one physician stepped in to defend me as "valiant," and another physician interjected that the thread had become "contentious."

An editor at Doximity who had been monitoring the exchange (perhaps alerted to it?) stepped in and apparently prevented one of the physicians from posting any more comments. (Doximity reserves the right to remove content it deems inappropriate.) It was reaffirming to receive a personal email from the Doximity editor informing me: "Your replies were, across the board, even-handed, professional, and respectful."

I've seen thousands of conversations exchanged online, and while the overwhelming majority of them are cordial and respectful, some of them are hostile, aggressive, and downright mean-spirited. To make matters worse, despite vigilant screening, Doximity and other medical websites allowed COVID disinformation to be published — by doctors of all people!

No one can ever guarantee that individuals who react to opinion pieces posted on a website will be courteous or professional. Every author takes a risk by publishing — indeed, *any* author on *any* platform opens themselves up to backlash and criticism by expanding their voice. But once again, the amount of rancor that prevails on medically oriented social media websites is disturbing and uncivil and possibly unethical at times.

Physicians as a group have become increasingly irritable and angry, and it shows not only in social media, but also in day-to-day interactions with patients. Stories of incivility abound. Your doctor was brusque because she couldn't pinpoint your problem (leaving you to feel it's all in your head). He rolls his eyes when you ask him for help (he's incapable of providing assistance). She becomes intolerant of your questions, stating, "We've covered this ground before" (she doesn't have time for you). He becomes petulant because you want a second opinion before surgery (he thinks he knows it all). She calls you "non-compliant" because you've stopped your medication (due to side effects). You're terminated from the practice without cause or due process.

While roughly 10% of all professions report disruptive behaviors, the number is higher in healthcare — about 30% . I have researched what ails American healthcare workers, especially physicians, and I have read myriad explanations as to why their behavior is so ornery. Most explanations can be summed up under the headings of stress and loss of autonomy — more than 50% of the physician workforce is now employed. Add to that a "cut-throat" culture that begins in college and carries through into medical school, where additional characteristics of the learning environment (e.g., negative role modelling, a stressful workload and an unbalanced focus on the biomedical model of disease [essay 34]) lead to loss of empathy, burnout, and career regret *by the time of graduation* in many cases, and you have a recipe for producing some of the most damaged, unhappy, miserable people on the planet — and they take out their frustrations on patients and each other.

I have read editorials that have suggested that social media platforms that promote extremist views and don't crack down on problematic content should be shut down. I think this is too drastic. Instead, I propose that habitually offending physicians be banned on social media until they take a qualified course in civility and communication to ensure they conduct themselves in the same professional manner as they would — or should — offline in a professional medical setting. Civility and professional communication practices are instrumental in attaining greater meaning in work, reducing frustration, and counteracting feelings of burnout, which might go a long way toward toning down doctors' online hubris and rhetoric.

Physicians Attacking Physicians Online: Trauma of the Second Order

When physicians take to the internet to discuss highly charged, potentially traumatic experiences they've encountered in practice, they risk being further traumatized by their colleagues' attacks — a brutal form of online "piling on."

THERE IS A TYPE OF ANNIVERSARY some of us in the medical profession commemorate because it reminds us of a traumatic experience we suffered sometime earlier in our career, often as a medical student or resident, when we were the "second" victims of trauma, also referred to as vicarious trauma. We are reminded of this trauma around the same time every year in the form of an "anniversary reaction."

I became interested in this topic because I was a victim myself — I suffered considerable anxiety and depression after a patient's suicide attempt during my first year of residency. The emotional repercussions were so severe they nearly caused me to leave. I researched vicarious trauma in healthcare providers and found that certain physicians were at higher risk of suffering psychiatric sequelae of trauma related to death, medical error, malpractice litigation, and other stressors encountered in practice.

Vicarious trauma is also a well-known occupational phenomenon for people working and volunteering outside of medicine in the fields of social services, law enforcement, fire services, and other professions, due to their continuous exposure to victims of trauma and violence. Individuals in those occupations suffer an outcome similar to physicians, with consequences ranging from burnout to depression to PTSD. Although the *Diagnostic and Statistical Manual of Mental Disorders* (DSM-5-TR) does not single out events related to medical practice, it does recognize "repeated or extreme indirect exposure to aversive details of a traumatic event" as a qualifying stressor sufficient to cause PTSD.

Yet, the prevailing medical culture seems to deter physicians from effectively dealing with the challenging emotions that naturally arise when confronted by patients facing death, trauma, accidents, and life-threatening illnesses — never mind bearing witness to human suffering in general. This was especially demoralizing during the pandemic. As an avid medical blogger, I have read many callous and unsympathetic remarks aimed at physicians seeking support and therapeutic relief by sharing their traumatic experiences online.

In one account, for example, an infectious disease specialist shared that she gave a patient with an ominous pulmonary infection the best possible care, yet the patient died — not an uncommon experience for doctors. While the overwhelming majority of readers' reactions were supportive and praiseworthy, one physician, a psychiatrist no less, was harsh and critical of the doctor, opining she did only "a minimal average acceptable job … [with] no clue whatsoever if the standard of care was met."

The psychiatrist also condemned me in one of my essays, insinuating that I had financial or other conflicts of interest simply for recommending that primary care physicians use mental health screening tools in their practice — screening instruments that are in the public domain, for which I receive no compensation. He was rude to another physician author who wrote an article discussing several ways physicians can supplement their income. The psychiatrist dismissed the article as "utterly useless."

In researching this psychiatrist's background, I found no original compositions penned by him. He is what we refer to in the vernacular as an internet "troll": a person who posts inflammatory, insincere, disruptive, digressive, extraneous, or off-topic messages in an online community. There is no place for trolls in a therapeutic — or any other — community.

Some of my most heartfelt editorials have been the target of uncivil physicians, as I mentioned in the preceding essay. I found myself at a war of words with a few colleagues whom I knew only by their online profiles. In several instances, I had to notify the editors of blogs that I believed these physicians' remarks constituted infractions of community standards, and I asked that the offending comments be removed (sometimes they were). Aggressive, unwarranted character attacks compound any past trauma physicians may be trying to overcome by off-loading their emotions in writing. Hostile and loathsome comments designed to undermine a physician's integrity are unprofessional and unwelcome, to say the least.

Even playful remarks made in jest may be viewed as taunting and teasing. When one such comment was directed my way, the commenter was taken to task by a community peer, who defended me and replied to the physician, "I must say that among your many comments that I encounter on[line], you always seem to find some way to poke your fellow clinicians' egos."

Rule number one when posting online is that comments should be phrased so as to foster productive and meaningful conversations with other community members. It's axiomatic that if you can't say anything nice, don't say anything at all.

When physicians write about upsetting experiences they've encountered in the course of clinical practice and share their stories online, they often seek solace and redemption through a community of like-minded peers. Narrative writing about medicine catalyzes a much-needed conversation about professional grief and trauma by including thoughtful essays (and poems), writing prompts, and community responses and discussion. Most physicians are sincere in their comments, but there are few bad actors who are unforgiving and unprofessional. They add another layer of burden to physicians already predisposed to stress, vulnerable to trauma, and possibly dealing with it.

It is well known that secondary exposure to patients' trauma can negatively affect the quality of care and professional well-being. Let's not also incorporate our fellow physicians' behavior into that mix of trauma. Physicians need to constructively engage with each other lest they begin to internalize their trauma, stop writing (or speaking), and continue to suffer in silence.

ESSAY 4

My Biggest Blind Spot Is Me

We all have "blind spots" — holes in our psyches that result in biases and prejudices. Patients and colleagues occasionally point them out. Clinical insight gleaned through practice also helps eliminate blind spots.

I TEND TO SIZE PEOPLE UP PRETTY QUICKLY. Adult ADHD? I can diagnose it in about two minutes. Borderline personality disorder? About one minute. Sociopaths on the Dr. Phil show? About 30 seconds (with the benefit of Dr. Phil's preamble). I can't help it. I attribute my habit of analyzing people to my training and practice in psychiatry. After a 40-year career in medicine, I can no longer delineate the psychiatrist from the private citizen. I don't even try.

Physicians occupy a lofty perch in society, or at least they used to. Given their status and power, their transactions with people tend to be one-sided. Until social media arrived on the scene, doctors rarely received feedback about themselves. One of my mentors, the subject of essay 38, founded a utilization review company in the 1980s and was so bold as to name it TAO (pronounced T-A-O). The acronym stood for transaction organization. Naturally, the transaction flowed irreversibly from the doctor to the patient.

When I was a resident, I discovered a lot about myself. Psycho-therapy was all but mandatory for psychiatric residents. This was fortunate, because therapy provided me insight and allowed me to adapt my persona to a range of patients with varying psycho-pathology. Still, due to the unilateral nature of the doctor-patient relationship, I felt beyond reproach. Also, as a psychiatrist, I could write off any interpretation about my behavior as "transference." I could simply inform my patients they were misdirecting their unconscious feelings and desires retained from childhood, which only strengthened my defenses and made me more impervious to other people's views of me.

My pomposity was eventually exposed by a patient. I thought the initial session went quite well, and I offered her the standard line, "Same time, next week?" She paused and replied, "I don't think I can see you again." I was puzzled and inquired further. "Look at your plants," she said, pointing to several of them wilting in my office, in desperate need of water. "If you can't take care of your plants, how do you expect to take care of me!"

Thank goodness there were additional people in my life who gave me accurate feedback about how I came across to them, about behaviors I wasn't aware of, my so-called blind spots. Sensitivity to others was once considered a prerequisite for a career in medicine. Somewhere along the way, in some of us, soft skills (described in essay 39) have taken a back seat to hard skills that enable us to endure medical training and the daily challenges of our profession, such as competitiveness, perfectionism, and other "type A" traits. Medical training often comes at the expense of compassion and empathy, and we tend to over-compensate for our emotional deficits by elevating ourselves above our patients.

As reviewed in the preceding two essays, medical bloggers who commented on my op-eds have given me a great deal of personal feedback, and they usually don't sugarcoat their remarks. When I bemoaned the lack of professional courtesy customarily accorded physicians and their families (essay 44), some physicians claimed I was entitled. When I wrote in the opening essay that proving other people wrong can sometimes be a source of motivation to succeed — a strategy I used to gain acceptance into medical school — a physician replied that he "pitied" me. Another physician commented that proving others wrong initially demonstrated that I did not have what it takes to succeed in life: ambition, motivation, and perseverance. And when I wrote about some of my experiences working for health-care organizations, specifically my fear of speaking out against my employer (essay 62), one physician commented, "Dr. Lazarus, you did it to yourself. You sacrificed your independence for a paycheck and became a proletariat."

While hard-hitting comments from colleagues were difficult to swallow and I tended to dismiss them, I knew those comments deserved my attention. It is well known that physicians have blind spots to the business of medicine, especially their employment contract options, but it is rarely appreciated that people from all walks of life know a significant amount about us yet we are in the dark. Many physicians recognize when their patients are noncompliant with treatment, but they may be incapable of recognizing faults in their own behavior. Common blind spots in physicians include:

- Cutting patients off before they are finished speaking.
- Lecturing patients without letting them get a word in.
- Multitasking when they should be listening.

Doctors with large blind spots have very little insight about themselves and their impact on patients. They may be able to make decisions and act quickly, but with little concern for the effect of their actions, and even less thought given to introspection. On the other hand, doctors with relatively small blind spots are practiced at noticing things about themselves and have a good bedside manner. It is important for physicians to connect the insight they have about themselves with the self-awareness they have gleaned from their patients and colleagues in order to maintain a balanced perspective on patient care.

I shared the content of some of my contentious online exchanges with a colleague. He nodded knowingly. "My biggest blind spot," he jokingly remarked, "is me."

Job Crisis: The Opportunity of a Lifetime

Every cloud has a silver lining. Learn how to recognize the opportunity present in the midst of a job crisis.

THE CHINESE WORD FOR "CRISIS" contains two elements: danger and opportunity. No matter the difficulty of circumstances, no matter how dangerous the situation, at the heart of every crisis there is a tremendous opportunity. It is said that great blessings lie ahead for the one who knows the secret of finding opportunity within each crisis.

I suppose I have been blessed many times over, because I have encountered crises of significant proportion throughout my career — not merely the mini-crises associated with putting out day-to-day fires, but rather the type of crisis that threatens your job security and makes you weak in the knees. Examples include:

- Serious adverse patient event/outcome.
- Job elimination.
- New boss.
- Change in executive leadership/governance.
- Relocation.
- Merger.
- Downsizing.
- Acquisition.
- Department of Justice investigation.

Each time I looked for the opportunity inherent in the crisis, I seemed to find it, although not right away and not without considerable introspection and anguish. Sometimes the outcome meant departing an organization for another job.

My first career crisis came during my initial year of residency in psychiatry. I touched on it in essay 3. Briefly summarized, while "on-call" one night, I made a treatment recommendation over the phone to another resident who had seen a schizophrenic patient in the emergency room (ER). I was not asked to evaluate the patient, so I simply told the ER doctor what I would do to treat the patient's "voices." The patient was discharged from the ER, but several hours later he returned, this time with two broken legs and other severe injuries sustained in a suicide attempt (he jumped from a third story window of his boarding home). I was devastated by the incident, and I berated myself for not going to the ER and doing the evaluation myself.

A crisis of confidence quickly set in. I doubted my skills and judgment, and I contemplated leaving the residency program for a job in the pharmaceutical industry. After seeking counsel, however, I decided to remain in the training program, eventually becoming chief resident and a faculty member in the psychiatry department.

Several opportunities emerged from this situation. First and foremost, I vowed to become a better doctor and take a more hands-on approach to patient care. Second, I entered psychotherapy to learn how to cope better with uncertainty and risk inherent in clinical practice. Third, I was able to complete my residency — a prerequisite for board certification and career advancement — and secure my immediate future in academic medicine. Joining the faculty was a big confidence booster to my career.

Midway through my career, I experienced a crisis related to job relocation. In order to take a prestigious job, I had to relocate to another city. Knowing that mobility is key to growing and expanding one's career, I felt compelled to take the job.

Relocation affects entire families. When I opted for a different job 5 years later, everyone was "all in" except my son, who, at the time was entering his senior year of high school. He refused to move with us and begin twelfth grade in a new school in a new city (could you blame him?). My wife and I decided to make the move with our three younger children and leave my son behind to finish his senior year.

We rented him a two bedroom, furnished, "corporate" apartment a short distance from his high school, and we bought him a used

Toyota Corolla to travel back and forth to school. We pretended he was a freshman in college rather than a senior in high school. Despite our trepidation, my son did not disappoint us. In fact, he has thanked us many times for placing our trust in him and emancipating him!

My most difficult job crisis occurred in 2001, the first time in my career my position was eliminated. My termination was not for cause. Still, I was given no option other than to leave the organization, a large health insurance company where I was VP and corporate medical director. I could not see any opportunity stemming from this harsh sentence, not even after reading the article *Congratulations… You're Fired!*, which was published just one year earlier in the *Physician Executive Journal* (July/August 2000), now the *Physician Leadership Journal.*

However, because I was allowed to stay with the company for one month after my initial notification, I had time to network for another job. Before my employment came to an end, I landed a job in the pharmaceutical industry. Talk about delayed gratification — 18 years had passed since I first considered a job in that industry! What you think may be a lost opportunity by giving up a job may circle back to you in the future.

I do not think I would have worked in "pharma" had my job at the health insurance company not been eliminated. My termination constituted another hidden opportunity. I worked for three pharmaceutical companies over the next 13 years. It was truly a wonderful experience. I did everything from clinical research to reviewing advertising and promotion for medical accuracy, as described in essay 42.

But once again I fell victim to organizational changes. In April 2014, my position as senior medical director at a pharmaceutical company was slated for elimination. I was given an opportunity stay on board as long as I was willing to accept a demotion to medical director and different responsibilities.

I was aware of the possible change to my position long before any changes were actually implemented, so I began a job search well before my position was impacted. I reconnected with a former employer. Paraphrasing Bob Dylan, it was a simple twist of fate that brought us back together. The opportunity that came with my new job, apart from the job itself, was the ability to relocate to Florida, which was a late-life goal.

Many people believe things happen for a reason. I can't say I relished all these job changes, or that I knew things would work out for the best. But in retrospect, they did. The opportunity embedded in a crisis at work is not always apparent. But having lived through many, I can say with relative certainty that the panic and fear related to a crisis, especially the ordeal of finding another job, lessens with each successive crisis.

Surviving Annual Performance Reviews

Performance evaluations are a fact of life, especially in large healthcare organizations. If you proactively manage the process, your chances of having a successful year will increase, and the stress and anxiety that accompany performance reviews will decrease.

PERFORMANCE MANAGEMENT IS A KEY PROCESS that enables organizations to function at their most competitive level. Executives must ensure that goals are clearly communicated throughout the organization, and that employees receive ongoing and actionable feedback with appropriate rewards and consequences. Since most physicians are now employed by healthcare organizations, they are not immune from having their performance evaluated.

But driving a high-performance culture in healthcare can be difficult because physicians often resist attempts to have their performance measured. They may be skeptical about how the evaluation will be used, and they frequently doubt the validity of the process itself. Physicians who once practiced independently and now work for large health systems are likely to view the review as unnecessary, if not an intrusion into practice.

Performance evaluations tend to provoke anxiety. They can be particularly stressful due to the high degree of rigor and conformity typical of large corporations, as well as the need to demonstrate to the public and investors a high performance and ethical culture. To survive annual performance reviews, keep these few points in mind.

Establish Measurable Goals and Outcomes

Create both short-term and long-term "SMART" goals — goals that are specific, measurable, attainable, realistic, and timely. Your goals and objectives should be aligned with the overall goals and objectives of your organization. Your company may have a "balanced scorecard" to help you identify key strategic priorities and provide a framework for measuring and carrying out your performance plan. Don't forget to identify development objectives that will be achieved over the coming year. It is important to get your boss to agree with your goals and objectives, preferably in writing.

Do Your Job Extremely Well

It is naïve to think you can do a lackluster job all year and escape scrutiny by your boss and coworkers. People observe you all the time and talk behind your back. Complaints about your performance may be lodged formally or informally. The only way to prevent them is to excel in your work and demonstrate a superlative work ethic. Apart from doing the technical aspects of your job well, you will be expected to exemplify the core values of your organization, demonstrate leadership, and deliver results that move the business forward.

Obtain Ongoing Feedback

In most large organizations, one or two formal feedback reviews — at interim and year-end — are the norm. Request feedback on your areas of strength and invite comments regarding opportunities for improvement. Many organizations employ a 360-degree feedback process at year-end to accomplish this feat. The feedback would come from subordinates, peers, and managers in your organization, and in some cases from external sources such as customers and interested stakeholders. You should provide a list of colleagues who know you well and can give candid responses. Avoid gaming the system by selecting only those individuals who are likely to give positive feedback about you.

Obtain Formal Mentoring When Necessary

Formal mentoring lies on a continuum between in-formal mentoring and coaching. Many organizations are implementing formal mentoring programs that, compared with informal mentoring described in essay 37, entail greater focus on developmental activities. Formal mentoring relationships pair mentees (often newly minted physicians) with senior leaders in the organization (not outside coaches). Mentees are exposed to effective learning experiences that help them grow and reach their objectives.

Learn to "Manage Up"

One of the most critical dimensions of performance management is the ability to manage upward. Managing up entails communicating effectively with your boss and other executives, and creating and maintaining strong bonds with them. Show them that you support their agenda and that they can count on your commitment and competence. By learning to discern the proper approach to take with your superiors, you can ensure that you are in the best position to gain from organizational opportunities that arise. Keep in mind that the art of managing upward should not be confused with "kissing up" or manipulating the system.

Collect Praise for Your Performance Throughout the Year

You will likely receive e-mail and other correspondence praising your performance throughout the year — perhaps a keynote address you gave, a visit to an important customer, or key insights shared with others. Acknowledgments for going the extra mile comprise an important component of your overall feedback, especially when the praise you receive is unsolicited. Save these e-mails and share them with your boss *before* they have completed your year-end evaluation.

Conduct All Performance Reviews In Person

Both the interim and year-end performance evaluations should be conducted face-to-face with your boss. Have a mid-year "sit-down" conversation with your boss to determine whether you are tracking against your goals and objectives and identify mechanisms to improve performance gaps. At the end of the year, a face-to-face meeting is necessary to determine your performance relative to your peers and business outcomes. Only through a private one-on-one meeting with your boss can the two of you explore what you accomplished and whether your objectives were met.

Sign Your Annual Performance Evaluation

Your signature on the year-end performance evaluation indicates that you have read it and accept it. If you have followed the steps outlined above, there should be no surprises. Let your boss know if you agree with your evaluation, and in the case of a disagreement, discuss options to remedy the situation. You may be able to persuade your boss to rewrite portions of the evaluation or reconsider issues related to compensation.

If you are highly dissatisfied with the evaluation and it cannot be changed, talk to someone in human resources. Ask if you can write an "addendum" to your evaluation, citing objective evidence that you believe would warrant a better evaluation than the one you received.

When Retirement Is Code for "You're Fired!"

Unless your retirement is for real, it's better to be honest with people and let them know what actually happened to cause you to lose your job. You needn't go into detail; a simple explanation will suffice, and you can spin it your way to save face.

A COLLEAGUE ANNOUNCES HE IS RETIRING.

Unknown to others at the time, there was a series of fires and suicides committed by patients at the psychiatric facility where he was chief medical officer during the year prior to his departure. State investigators condemned the incidents and found an array of policy failures and procedural errors compounded by staffing shortages due to the coronavirus pandemic.

Another colleague announces his retirement. Unknown to others at the time, the health insurance company where he is chief medical officer is hemorrhaging cash. The insurer is negotiating with a larger company to be acquired. The chief medical officer is blamed, in part, for the poor financial performance of his department, and he is considered expendable during the merger.

In the months leading up to the merger, several of the company's medical directors are dismissed in a last-ditch effort to stop the bleeding. I am one of those medical directors. I announce my retirement.

The late Howard Kirz, MD, wrote: "Being fired as a physician executive is the dark side of burgeoning opportunities for health care leadership. The risk of termination is 20 to 40 times higher than for clinicians." He found that almost 50% of physician executives will involuntarily lose their jobs within five years of being hired. Reasons include: organizational restructuring, financial losses, new or unclear responsibilities, conflict with a boss or board member, and ineffective leadership. In addition, physicians embroiled in medico-legal investigations and litigation have been engulfed by the winds of change.

Some Scrooge-like employers have been known to fire long-time employees — some with decades of loyal service under their belt — just before they were eligible to retire and collect a pension or other benefits. Publicly traded healthcare companies have awarded physicians stock or stock options as an incentive to retain them, only to let them go before the stock has vested. Employers may or may not give physicians the ability to develop an exit strategy and save face upon termination.

When confronted with a forced job severance, the first question to ask yourself is this: Do you want to take this opportunity to retire, or do you prefer to continue working (elsewhere, of course)?

Hopefully, if you truly want to retire, you've planned for this day.

If you want to continue working, it is probably best to inform your colleagues you are leaving for "personal reasons" rather than make an insincere declaration about retiring.

There are several other ways to finesse the reason for your unplanned departure without resorting to the retirement cliché. Savvy coworkers understand that "retirement" is often a code word for "fired." Your retirement announcement may invite all kinds of questions you may not be prepared to answer or simply do not (or cannot) care to discuss.

Do you think my psychiatrist friend wanted to explain that an investigative panel held him (and others) accountable for shoddy conditions that led to two fires and three suicide deaths inside the hospital he oversaw? Do you think he wanted the story and his name plastered on the front page of the local newspaper six months after his "retirement" so that everyone could discover the truth behind his leaving?

The fact is only about 50 to 60 suicides take place among hospital inpatients every year in the United States. Three cases in the same institution in a nine-month span is not an anomaly. The embarrassment, guilt, and shame that are likely to emerge in a physician thus compromised can become crippling and demoralizing. No one wants to suffer this fate late in their career.

Do you think my boss who worked for the faltering health insurance company really wanted to explain how he was held accountable (scapegoated?) for factors beyond his control — factors that had more to do with market conditions and unrealistic organizational goals — and that such factors often result in the downfall of physician executives?

That's why when it became my time to announce my retirement, I really meant it. (I had a change of heart a year later and decided to work part-time.)

According to a 24-year study by ProPublica and the Urban Institute, there is a 56% chance that workers over age 50 will be let go before they're ready to retire, risking substantial income loss.

So, assuming you plan on working into your late 50s, 60s, and 70s, it's likely the ax will fall on you at least one time.

Do not disguise your job termination as a retirement. Furthermore, on your way out, determine whether you can negotiate a severance package with your employer. Here are a few things to consider as you transition to your next job:

1. Maximize your network and keep your skills — especially technology — cutting edge.
2. Agree on the "parting line" and obtain a positive reference — in writing — from your boss or someone in a leadership position.
3. Collect favorable performance reviews you've received.
4. Gather contact information from coworkers who can serve as future references.
5. Develop a powerful "pitch" for potential employers, one that demonstrates your value.
6. Play an active role in structuring your next position.
7. Leave in style. Never trash your employer to future employers.

When it comes time to retire for good, without a hidden agenda or the possibility of anyone misinterpreting your reasons for leaving, don't announce your retirement too early. Ironically, you can be fired after announcing your plans to retire. Many physicians feel the need to give advance notice so their employer can find a replacement, and that's a great sentiment. But sentiment and business rarely mix.

Besides, most likely, you will have been employed "at will," which means you can be terminated at any time, with or without cause. Thus, you shouldn't feel compelled to give advance notice unless you are contractually obligated to do so. If you really want to give several months' notice, wait until it won't hurt you financially in case your employer opts for immediate termination.

No matter what the circumstance surrounding your job termination, don't take your firing personally. Think of yourself as a recovering taxpayer until something new comes along. Beware, however, that the ProPublica and the Urban Institute study revealed that only about 10% of workers went on to earn comparable salaries at another job. It also took them much longer — a year or more — to find another job than their younger counterparts (see essay 12)

The bottom line: Make sure your retirement announcement is not a cover-up for losing a job. Losing a job anytime in your career can be traumatic. But it doesn't mean that your days in the workforce are numbered. You just have to use your skills, experience, and knowledge and search harder to find another job. It worked for me. It will work for you.

Is Your Medical Specialty Sustainable?

As you think about your current or intended specialty, visualize its future and how it will impact your practice and career satisfaction. If the picture appears bleak, consider a specialty that adds variety to your practice.

MEDICAL STUDENTS' SELECTION OF A SPECIALTY is one of the most important choices they will ever make. But the decision about which medical specialty to enter can be difficult for many students. One of the difficulties lies in the fact that it is impossible for students to sample all their options while in medical school (approximately 20 specialties in total, not including subspecialties), let alone determine the ideal location to undertake training — assuming they match to their first choice.

Another reason choosing a specialty may be problematic is that the fields of medicine change over time. My specialty of psychiatry, for example, was founded on the principles of psychotherapy — psychoanalysis in particular. But the provision of outpatient psychotherapy by U.S. psychiatrists has declined significantly over the past two decades. In the 2010s, about half of psychiatrists did not incorporate psychotherapy into their practice, yet psychotherapy training continues to be required by psychiatric residency programs in order to maintain accreditation.

To choose a specialty, medical students need to think like Wayne Gretzky, considered the greatest hockey player of all time. When asked how he managed to play so well and score so many goals, Gretzky said he skated to where he thought the puck was going to be, not where it was. By focusing on the future — where the puck is going to be — students can set themselves up to remain ahead of the curve and enjoy a specialty that will hold their interest for a lifetime. Choosing a specialty with staying power can also help them avoid burnout.

I'm no Wayne Gretzky, but I did tend to think like him when it came time to choose my specialty. I majored in psychology in college, and I always had an interest in the relationship between the brain and behavior. In my final year of medical school, I was well aware that the field of psychiatry was loosening its grip on psychotherapy and gravitating to an understanding of the biological basis of behavior. In hockey terms, my specialty choice was based on where I thought the puck was going to be, i.e., where the field of medicine was trending, particularly the practice of psychiatry.

There is an underlying assumption in Gretzky's quote: We can predict an outcome (where the puck is going to be) based on the detection of certain signals (where the puck is and what is happening at the time). To ensure I had a full view of the hockey arena, I consulted one of my mentors — a neurologist. I was equally as interested in neurology as I was in psychiatry, and I vacillated between the two disciplines.

I shared my dilemma with my mentor, and he replied, "Well, Art, if you want my opinion, one day, psychiatry will become a subspecialty of neurology." The neurologist's forward-looking prediction did not come true — at least not yet — but it is a fact that we now consider serious mental illnesses the equivalent of brain disorders, and both neurology and psychiatry have long been governed by the same Board of the American Board of Medical Specialties — namely, the American Board of Psychiatry and Neurology.

Today, the landscape of medicine looks vastly different than it did when I trained in the 1980s. Back then, artificial intelligence, telehealth, genetics and gene editing, and concierge and integrative medical practices were barely on the horizon, if at all. In my eventual area of specialization — pharmaceutical medicine — clinical trials were conducted at the site of the principal investigator, usually an academic medical center. Nowadays, decentralized clinical trials are the big rave. We are in the process of enabling clinical trials to be conducted at the home of subjects, much like making house calls. Decentralized trials aid in the recruitment and retention of subjects, increase the speed of the trial and diversity of subjects, and facilitate data collection.

Whether in practice or in industry, predicting how clinical scenarios will unfold is key to choosing where and how you may want to spend your working time. Unfortunately, critical areas of medicine are often the least satisfying specialties because advances in those fields tend to occur at a slow pace. On the other hand, specialties perceived to be dynamic and rapidly changing, and that offer a diversity of work, often provide the greatest personal fulfillment. You do have to do your homework and consider whether a given specialty is likely to innovate or remain stagnant.

As I previously mentioned, consulting with mentors — often academic faculty — can help you arrive at a decision. Ironically, in my case, a physician who was not a specialist in my field influenced my decision. But just to be certain he had guided me in the right direction, I sought the advice of a well-known psychiatrist on staff at my medical school. I told him what the neurologist had said about how psychiatry is becoming absorbed by neurology. The psychiatrist paused and commented, "No, Art. The neurologist is wrong. Tell him one day psychiatry will become a subspecialty of toxicology."

I think they were both correct!

The "Golden Consult" Revisited

Hierarchies and power imbalances are prevalent throughout the medical field, even among physicians who hold the same academic rank. Disparities between specialists often surface around clinical consultations.

For years, scholars have thought the perfect surgery consult was impossible. Comedic ophthalmologist Will Flanary, a.k.a. Dr. Glaucomflecken, characterizes the golden consult as one in which the surgeon is not consulted too soon — because the patient is not sick enough to require their services — and one in which the surgeon is not consulted too late, or else the patient may die.

For a consult to be "golden," timing is everything. In addition, the length of the consult matters. If the consult is too long, the surgeon will lose interest, and the patient will be shuffled off to the medical service. If the consult is too short — one word, for example — an orthopedic surgeon will be called in.

The real-life Dr. Will Flanary knows quite a bit about surgery because he is a survivor of recurrent testicular cancer. His admirers — 2.5 million subscribers across TikTok, YouTube, and Twitter — claim he brings truth to stark medical realities while poking fun at his colleagues and the profession, nudging doctors away from what can be a monastic self-regard.

Dr. Glaucomflecken's take on surgical consults got me thinking about the relationship between surgeons and psychiatrists. Psychiatrists don't often consult surgeons, but I did so twice during my PGY-1 residency year. The first time was for a newly admitted psychotic woman. When her lab values came back indicating thyrotoxicosis, the surgeons whisked her away for subtotal thyroidectomy. It was the quickest cure for psychosis I had ever witnessed.

The second consult was not so golden. It was for a woman who had been struggling against restraints while psychotic and began complaining of arm pain as her psychosis (due to benzodiazepine withdrawal) resolved. An orthopedic resident diagnosed frozen shoulder and recommended "aggressive PT." There was no review of the case by an attending surgeon.

The actual diagnosis was bilateral humeral fracture/dislocation, uncovered months after the patient was discharged from the hospital — too late for surgical intervention. The patient suffered chronic pain and eventually died by suicide. Her children initiated a lawsuit against the hospital and all doctors involved in her care, including me.

The name of the orthopedic resident was never known — his name was illegible on the consultation form, and he had completed his residency and left the institution for private practice. The complaint listed the orthopedic resident as a John Doe. A settlement was reached prior to trial. I don't think I ever consulted a surgeon again.

However, I performed many consultations as a psychiatrist working on an academic consultation-liaison service. Like Dr. Glaucomflecken, I believed there was such a thing as a "golden consult." For psychiatrists, it was one in which the referring physician understood the gravity of the patient's psychiatric condition and the criteria for inpatient hospitalization. The admission should not be requested for convenience, a social disposition problem, delirium, dementia or a combative or unruly medical patient.

Physicians possess varying levels of expertise depending on their areas of specialization. Specialization drives differences in diagnostic practice and creates a clinical imbalance that may cause some of us to have a jaundiced view of our colleagues.

We all have our own notion of what constitutes the golden consult — from our own perspective, of course. Treatment disagreements and turf wars often result from disparities in our medical sophistication — our depth of knowledge and ability to understand clinical nuances. The consultant's knowledge obviously runs deeper than the consultee's. Why else would a consultation be requested?

I was consulted by a surgeon when I was chief resident. Although I was accustomed to physicians dumping patients in our psych unit, the opposite situation now presented itself. A prominent head-and-neck surgeon refused to have his patient admitted to our inpatient psychiatry unit after his patient had attempted suicide. The patient tried to asphyxiate himself because he could no longer bare the disfigurement caused by extensive surgery for oral cancer.

To make matters worse, the surgeon was the father of one of my medical school classmates. He actually taught us the anatomy of the neck on our cadaver during our freshman year. He did not remember me now, nearly eight years hence, but I surely remembered him. I was able to convince the surgeon that his patient would be better served in the psych unit, where we could thoroughly evaluate his mental status and institute treatment to improve his self-esteem, all in a setting of safety.

Both the surgeon and the patient consented to treatment, and the patient was discharged in much better spirits without suicidal ideation.

Most of what I've read about power asymmetry in medicine has addressed the dynamic between doctors and patients and how it prevents shared decision-making. However, understanding the power hierarchy among physicians is equally important, and for the same reason: it skews treatment decisions in the direction of the powerful. Apart from one's area of specialization, numerous sources contribute to conflict and imbalance of power between physicians, such as differences in training levels (e.g., medical student versus resident versus attending), gender, race, and ethnicity, particularly as they impact black women in medicine.

Power imbalances among physicians often surface around consultations. Perhaps joking about it is one way of dealing with it; however, given that power imbalances can become toxic and destroy the workplace experience for many physicians, residency programs and healthcare systems must look carefully at the wide-ranging consequences of tolerating and rewarding the unacceptable behavior of high-performing physicians at the expense of trainees, staff, and the medical community.

It's been said that "Flanary's best material balances the specificity of an expert with the nose for hypocrisy that typically comes from an incisive observer." Shouldn't we all pay closer attention to the way we treat each other and avoid microaggressions and other demeaning and hurtful remarks, even if we believe (erroneously) that power permits us to take such liberties? If we're going to talk in jest about inequities in medicine, shouldn't we all be in on the joke?

Call Me In, Not Out, For My Transgressions

Microaggressions permeate medical practice and have widespread consequences for physicians and patients. It's best to call physicians "in," not "out," to make them aware of their prejudices. Those who continue to behave badly should be required to undergo education and sensitivity training at the very least.

I LOST MY PATIENCE when the food-delivery driver called me and said she could not find her way to our house. Our home is newly constructed and does not appear in some GPS systems. Sometimes GPS guides people to a location near where we live. Unfortunately, this malfunction includes the GPS system used by delivery drivers who work for a certain online food ordering company.

Although the driver was lost, she was in my neighborhood — I could tell because I recognized the names of the streets she was reading aloud as she drove past them. The driver's English was limited, which was somewhat unnerving. I was able to guide her to our home, but my tone was gruff, perhaps because she interrupted my viewing of the nightly news, or because I was "hangry" — our dinnertime meal was 25 minutes late. My anger also stemmed from the fact that I had quite a bit of difficulty communicating with her.

I met the driver at the curb, waving her down as she approached our house, in fear she might overshoot it. She stepped out of her compact car — a vehicle that had obviously seen better days — and handed over the meal. I composed myself and thanked her.

"Where do you come from," I asked?

"Ukraine," she replied.

My heart sank. I was suddenly ashamed of the way I had treated her over the phone. The nightly news that she interrupted? Lester

Holt was giving an update on casualties in Ukraine from extensive bombing that day.

"You know there's a problem with the GPS system you are using," I said in a conciliatory tone. "Here, let me show you a better app for directions," as I introduced her to "Waze" on my iPhone.

Now collected, I was less bothered by her meager English as she explained that online orders through the delivery app are automatically linked to their GPS system. However, she took note of the "Waze" application as a back-up and said she would use it in the future, if necessary.

I took our dinner inside, but I had lost my appetite. I couldn't come to terms with my initial unfriendliness. It was uncharacteristic of me. In my mind, there were inciting factors for the way I behaved, yet they were clearly based on prejudice and couldn't justify my disrespect of the driver or undo the interaction.

I became engulfed by my thoughts: Was I guilty of microaggressions with patients before I retired from practice? How many patients might I have offended or incensed due to biased thinking? Surely, I saw many patients who spoke English as a second language. Was I negatively predisposed to all of them?

I flashed back to my years spent in training and clinical practice in Philadelphia. The diversity of people living there enriched my education. English as a second language — or no English spoken — was never a problem. We had interpreters on staff. On one occasion (before HIPAA) I enlisted the corner hot dog vendor to help me translate for a patient who spoke only Greek.

I was outraged when Joseph ("Joey") Vento, the owner of Geno's Steaks, a local eatery and shrine, slapped a sign in the window declaring that only English-speaking customers would be served. It read: "This is AMERICA. When ordering, speak English." I protested by ordering from rival "Pat's King of Steaks" across the street. The sign attracted national attention, and legal attempts to remove it were unsuccessful. The sign was voluntarily removed in 2016, a decade after it was posted.

My thoughts also reverted to the 1970s and the era of Frank Rizzo, the former Philadelphia police commissioner turned mayor turned radio talk-show host. Rizzo was known widely for his racist and anti-gay views, leaving a legacy of unchecked police brutality.

The aggression exhibited by Vento and Rizzo was at the "macro" level. On the other hand, my emotional response to the driver delivering my food was more subtle — a microaggression. Microaggressions are flash-in-the-pan behaviors that stem from implicit biases toward people unlike us.

Implicit biases are unconscious stereotypes, assumptions, and beliefs held about an individual's identity. They affect our understanding, actions, and decisions, and increase health disparities. The important point is that implicit biases influence diagnoses and patient treatment even in the absence of a physician's intent or awareness, because ingrained biases are never truly extinguished — they leave a "mental residue."

Learning how to identify and overcome implicit biases is essential to improving the delivery of healthcare to diverse populations. The first step is to look for stereotyped descriptors in the electronic health record. A recent study found that, compared with white patients, black patients were two and a half times more likely to be described in negative terms, such as "non-compliant," "agitated," and "refused." The authors concluded that providers may not be able to change their belief systems without self-awareness and/or training on potential biases.

Such training may take the form of a patient-centered approach to cross-cultural care, cultural competency training, and other types of education aimed at recognizing stereotypical thinking. The key is to learn how to replace biases and assumptions with accurate representations of patients free of racial and ethnic context, and increase opportunities for positive contact with geographically and socioeconomically disadvantaged patients.

Loretta J. Ross, associate professor at Smith College, adds that when microaggressions occur, shaming people is a natural impulse but not necessarily the correct option. It is better to call people in rather than call them out, she says. Calling in is similar to calling out, but it's done privately and with respect. Calling in involves conversation, compassion, and context. Ross remarks, "...take comfort in the fact that you offered a new perspective of information and you did so with love and respect, and then you walk away..." The calling-in practice entails reserving a seat at the table for transgressors if, at first, they are not receptive to your kind gesture but later decide to join the conversation.

So, to all my former patients — and any other individuals I may have transgressed against — I humbly seek your forgiveness and ask that you call me in rather than call me out.

Like Many Physicians, I've Forgotten How to Relax

*Many physicians are wound up and tightly wired.
You would think something like a good vacation
would be a cure. But ironically, unchained from
their daily routine, achieving tranquility seems
impossible, even on a tropical island.*

Here I am, in January 2023, on vacation at a luxury resort in Hawaii with my wife and two of my four children and their three children. It's 10 p.m. and I'm beginning to write this essay while everyone is snug and tucked away for the night. Earlier in the day, sitting around the swimming pool, I was glued to my iPhone. My son, who resides in Honolulu, commented, "Dad, you're so wired in. Play with the kids (my grandchildren) in the splash zone. Take them on a ride down the lazy river. Relax with us."

But like many physicians, I've forgotten how to relax. Patient care has been front and center since the pandemic started — in addition to the usual crises and emergencies — and we're increasingly burned out or are using substances to cope. Our clinical performance has diminished, resulting in increased errors and other quality concerns.

The one thing we've been good at, it seems, is neglecting our own health. Researchers found that physicians who were wedded to their jobs experienced lower quality of sleep, greater levels of depression, and lower levels of general well-being. Plus, they exhibited more stress at work.

Everyone knows that doctors need to take time for themselves and relax in order to stay healthy. Providing doctors with opportunities to relax is correlated with better health outcomes for themselves and their patients. Trips to far-away or exotic locations can be helpful but are not guaranteed to afford relaxation. Sometimes simply walking 30 minutes each day, partaking in a hobby, meditating, and other pleasurable activities are all that is needed to recharge your batteries.

However, some doctors find it difficult to engage in relaxing activities. I admit, I'm one of them. I have a collection of several hundred concert DVDs; approximately half are unopened and waiting to be viewed. I've purchased dozens of books not yet read. What makes it difficult for doctors like me to sit down, relax, and watch a DVD or read a good book? The answer, according to experts, lies in our brain chemistry and conditioning.

Our brains want a dopamine rush, and our sympathetic nervous system is stuck in overdrive. Physicians rely on a steady diet of distressing news, disturbing deaths, and clinical disasters. After years of medical practice, excitement fades, replaced by boredom and panic. Our brains seek a quick chemical hit to rekindle. Rarely do we have a chance to debrief over critical incidents and reflect on what happened. We just move on, tense and stressed out, always in a hurry to "get to the point," bypassing important cognitive ramifications of our work.

In terms of conditioning, we've been primed, prepped, and propelled toward academic and career success since high school, perhaps earlier. Along the way, we've been challenged by automatic negative thoughts: "I'm going to flunk this test," "I can't handle the work load," "I don't measure up," "I'm an imposter." Automatic negative thoughts can result in fatigue, depression, anxiety, and symptoms typically associated with trauma, especially hyperarousal, which contributes to our inability to relax. Anyone who grew up thinking they had to be the "best" is likely programmed for stressful perfectionism incompatible with relaxation.

I first noticed my difficulty relaxing while in medical school. Absorbing the basic sciences was like taking a drink from the proverbial firehose: a tsunami of new information crashed upon me as soon as I felt up-to-date (see essay 29). During clinical rotations, I was anxious and on guard, waiting to be pimped by a senior resident or an attending. I invested energy in all clerkships. In reality, no specialty other than psychiatry appealed to me. I became chief psychiatry resident thanks to my unsurpassed achievements and devotion to training. However, the work involved "staying ahead" of my peers and precluded relaxation.

Once in practice, I thought my nerves would settle down, but they didn't. I read *The Relaxation Response*. The good advice in that book was offset by a personal, stressful mission to "find the way to myself" — the raison d'être espoused by Emil Sinclair, the protagonist in Hermann Hesse's *Demian*. Sinclair wanted to know why it was so difficult "to live in accord with the promptings which came from [his] true self." Our search for meaning is an exhaustive process, fraught with uncertainty and fear. How could anyone relax under those conditions?

Yet, I identified with Sinclair, especially the passage in *Demian* in which he realizes that "[man's] task was to discover his own destiny — not an arbitrary one — and to live it out wholly and resolutely within himself. Everything else was only a would-be existence, an attempt at evasion, a flight back to the ideals of the masses, conformity and fear of one's own inwardness." I certainly didn't want my existence to be "arbitrary."

So, I embarked on a journey of self-discovery with the help of a wise and compassionate psychoanalyst. He provided expert guidance for my travels. However, even after therapy, I was consumed by free-floating anxiety. I never felt totally relaxed, and even to this day, at a time when I consider myself semi-retired, I'm always looking over the horizon for the next challenge, the next big fix, the next accomplishment, the next op-ed to write.

Apparently, patience is not a virtue of many doctors. I've read stories about physicians in various specialties — not only psychiatry — who have struggled to relax when off work. Only 60% of doctors report feeling "happy" outside of work. Fortunately, some physicians have managed to compensate for their unhappiness and restlessness through extracurricular activities, as I discuss in essay 18 and as demonstrated in the following examples:

An emergency medicine physician finds bicycle riding a great way to decompress. He becomes "lost" in his thoughts as he rides, sometimes forgetting specifics along the route.

A family medicine physician turns to prayer and religion to relax. Other activities such as walking on nature trails and even sitting by the fireplace remind her there's more to life than practicing medicine.

An otolaryngologist who specializes in head and neck cancer surgery engages in outdoor activities like camping, boating, and fishing with his family. His stress is reduced by working with his hands, enjoying hobbies such as woodcarving and tinkering with cars.

A pulmonologist and critical care physician paints and makes craft projects with her son. Yoga and cooking are her favorite ways to unwind.

I'm thinking about leaving my computer and smart devices at home the next time I take a vacation. I informed my son of my intentions. He took me to his favorite coffee café. "Everyone's connected and engaged here," he said, pointing to a sign that read: "Sorry, No WiFi 4 U." A smile crossed my face. I began to relax.

Does Ageism Lurk Behind Mandatory Retirement for Physicians?

"The young man knows the rules, but the old man knows the exceptions." — Oliver Wendell Holmes

IN ESSAY 7, I related a story about a good friend and colleague — the chairman of a psychiatry department — who notified people he was retiring. In a department newsletter, he wrote, "I sent out a letter to the alumni and adjunct faculty that I will retire on June 30 [2021]. I had decided five years ago that when I reached a certain age, I was going to retire. Such decisions have multiple determinants and are made with ambivalent feelings."

My friend was on the faculty for 20 years and chairman for half that time. He further wrote, "It has been a wonderful journey. Watching many residents and faculty become outstanding clinicians, educators, and researchers has been an honor and joy. These wonderful relationships are part of the tapestry of my memory and will always remind me of my years at [the medical school]. I am leaving a vibrant, energetic, and young faculty."

"Why retire?" I thought. It didn't make sense that my friend would impose an age limit on himself to retire when he was 70 and cognitively intact. Sometime later I discovered that he had become embroiled in conflict with the university, and his departure had nothing to do with his age, competence, or views about his age.

Yet I know there are times when aging physicians begin to show signs of dementia and are singled out for neuropsychological evaluations. Similarly, some surgeons seem physically unfit to operate and are subjected to ophthalmological and neurological testing. In fact, this topic — the competency of older physicians to practice medicine — has become a raging controversy.

The issue concerns whether physicians should be forced to retire at a certain age like other professionals, such as judges, FBI agents, commercial pilots, air traffic controllers, military officers, and national park rangers. During her 2024 presidential campaign, former South Carolina Governor Nikki Haley called for mandatory competency tests for politicians older than 75. "In the America I see, the permanent politician will finally retire," Haley said — except most older voters balked at her idea.

The argument for mandatory retirement almost always centers on public safety. Older ("permanent") physicians are believed to threaten patients' safety because aging impacts not only cognition but also vision, hearing, dexterity, stamina, and judgment. A 2005 article in the *Annals of Internal Medicine* kicked off a firestorm when the authors reviewed 62 studies and found that more than half (52%) showed a decline in patient outcomes with advanced practitioner age (only one study showed improvement).

A 2017 study in the *British Medical Journal* offered further proof that aging results in errors and poorer quality care. Among hospitalists in charge of Medicare patients, older physicians had higher 30-day mortality rates than those cared for by younger physicians, despite similar patient characteristics. The only variable that resulted in comparable mortality rates was high patient volume, in which case, young or old, it didn't make a difference in patient mortality.

However, a 2021 analysis of 52 studies found quite the opposite, i.e., physicians' clinical experience (a proxy for age) and quality tended to be positively correlated. Moreover, in a study of surgeons, age was not an important predictor of operative risk, including mortality, for most procedures. In yet another study, residents and attendings were judged to be equal in their safety outcomes. A subsequent study of emergency medicine physicians found that older physicians fared better than younger ones in terms of committing fewer errors, prompting some to argue that training resources should be directed toward novice physicians instead of elderly ones.

Overall, the literature on this subject is complicated and conflicting, with marked variation in results and divided opinions about implementing mandatory competency testing or retirement for physicians, usually beginning at age 70.

Ageism is one significant factor that clouds findings and interpretations; it is the elephant in the room. The term "ageism" was coined in 1968 by psychiatrist Robert N. Butler (1927–2010), who became the first director of the National Institute on Aging. Butler, a fierce defender against discrimination and stereotypes of the elderly, compared ageism to racism, claiming it was "prejudice by one age group toward other age groups." (Butler did not discuss "reverse ageism" coming from older workers toward younger professionals.)

In one of his seminal papers, "Age-Ism: Another Form of Bigotry," Butler wrote: "Ageism reflects a deep-seated uneasiness on the part of the young and middle-aged — a personal revulsion to and distaste for growing old, disease, disability; fear of powerlessness, 'usefulness,' and death." I do not doubt that much of the controversy surrounding the mandatory retirement of physicians is rooted in ageism.

Nowhere is this more evident than in institutions embarking on late-career practitioner screening programs, notably Yale New Haven Hospital, which is tied up in litigation with the U.S. Equal Employment Opportunity Commission over attempts to evaluate physicians simply because they are old. At Yale and other institutions, it is quite possible that policies may reflect ageist attitudes rather than genuine concerns about patient safety, and that implicit (unconscious) bias may be at work — a type of microaggression toward the elderly.

A 2022 study from Switzerland bears this out. There was a tendency among 234 human resource (HR) employees to see themselves as less biased than their HR peers or to be able to identify more cognitive biases in others than in themselves in their hiring decisions. The presence of a biased "blind spot" was thus confirmed (see essay 4). Furthermore, male HR employees showed a greater bias blind spot than female HR employees.

Age bias is one of the most common types of discrimination in the workplace today. This is very concerning for physicians, given that approximately 47% of active physicians in the United States in 2021 were 55 or older, and some plan to practice until they are in their 70s or 80s. An age mandate to retire will deplete the physician workforce and wreak havoc on a system already facing dire shortages.

For sure, there are physicians advancing in age who should be removed from the workforce. There are also early-career physicians who should not be allowed to practice. Assessing physician competencies and capabilities based on identities like age and other demographics is only a hop-skip-and-a-jump away from using other factors like illness, gender, or race as cause for discriminatory policies disguised as "patient safety."

The solution is to target the performance of individual physicians when their abilities are in question, rather than target an entire class of physicians, and begin collecting normative data for various age groups to prevent judgments from being made in isolation.

The AMA Principles of Medical Ethics also propose a way to solve the conundrum of mandatory retirement. It recognizes that physicians have a duty to monitor the quality of care they deliver as individual practitioners, e.g., through personal case review and critical self-reflection, peer review, and the use of other quality improvement tools. Physicians are responsible for maintaining their health and wellness. When practice issues arise, take measures to mitigate them, seek appropriate help as necessary and engage in an honest self-assessment of their ability to continue practicing.

For example, Richard Rothman, MD (1936–2018), was one of the nation's most prominent and respected orthopedic surgeons. He was still doing surgery at age 80. However, he had his vision checked regularly and asked a senior partner to monitor the quality of his work for a day (he did fine). Rothman may have been a role model for the AMA, but how often can physicians be expected to follow his lead?

The Benefits of Facing Mortality

Mortality has motivational properties. Life becomes more precious as we near the end of it. We have to decide which activities are worth pursuing and which ones should be forsaken. One thing seems certain – I won't stop writing!

ACCORDING TO CHRIS JORDAN, a New Jersey shore native who writes about music and entertainment, Bruce Springsteen and the E Street Band performed "like their lives depended on it" when they kicked off their 2023 tour in Tampa, Florida, in early February. The tour kept the 73-year-old Springsteen on the road for six months, playing over 60 concerts, proving that mortality can be a motivating force resulting in increased productivity while also dismantling the myth that productivity decreases with age.

Not that "The Boss" is in imminent danger of dying. He seems quite fit, playing high-octane concerts lasting almost three hours. But considering that hardly a week goes by without news of the death of a rock star, when Springsteen plays a stripped-down version of "Last Man Standing" from his 2020 album, *Letter to You*, you begin to understand why death is on Springsteen's mind.

"Last Man Standing" is a reference to Springsteen, the last surviving member of his first group, The Castiles. Following the 2018 death of his Castiles bandmate George Theiss, Springsteen told *Rolling Stone* that Theiss' death sparked deep reflections on mortality and spurred him to write many of the tunes on *Letter to You*. Springsteen said to the concert-goers in Tampa: "[Mortality] brings a clarity of thought and a purpose that you might have not previously experienced. At 15, it's all tomorrows. At 73, it's a lot of goodbyes. That's why you have to make the most of right now." Springsteen replayed the song and the story in each of his 60+ concerts.

You don't have to be a baby boomer to relate to what Springsteen is saying, although boomers comprise 21.6% of the US population, and they are the main age group attending his concerts, including his long run on Broadway. Baby boomers are now (in 2023) between 59 and 77 years of age. About one-third of baby boomers have died. The "last man standing" of that generation will be gone by about 2086. What boomer doesn't have death on their mind?

Contemplating death is not necessarily bad. According to psychologist Steve Taylor, being more aware of your own mortality can be a positive development. He came to this conclusion while working on his book *Out of the Darkness* and after interviewing individuals with terminal illnesses, as well as people who have had near-death experiences, such as those who had a heart attack or almost drowned.

Taylor wrote: "Facing death had taught them that the future and the past are unimportant, and that life only ever takes place in the present moment.... Becoming aware of our own mortality can be a liberating and awakening experience, which can — paradoxically, it might seem — encourage us to live authentically and fully for the first time."

There are many great books about death and dying, such as *Being Mortal* and *With the End in Mind*. They describe how we should treat dying loved ones: gently, with dignity, compassion, forethought, and preparation. This message should never be lost upon us. However, I'm equally impressed by the notion that the sudden realization that our time on earth is limited not only instructs us to live in the moment but it also seems to enhance our productivity. And since physical activity improves virtually every health outcome, it offers the option of a longer, healthier life.

Springsteen isn't the only musician who understands that facing mortality may increase productivity. Country singer Willie Nelson commemorated turning 90 by winning a Grammy, hitting the road, and releasing another top-quality record ("I Don't Know A Thing About Love") — his 15th album in the past decade. Likewise, David Crosby lived to 81, and his final decade was his most productive.

In South Korea, some companies are using mock funerals as a way to combat employee depression and increase productivity. (South Korea has consistently had one of the highest suicide rates in the world.) After the employees emerge from wooden coffins in their pretend funerals, they allegedly have a better outlook on life and work, now that they have glimpsed the alternative.

I'm reminded of the relationship between mortality and productivity whenever I encounter people who have a "bucket list" — a list of activities to do before dying — that is, before "kicking the bucket." People on a mission to complete their bucket list are not necessarily terminally ill; a sizable percentage simply realize time is precious and they had better get moving.

I turned 69 in January 2023. I'm in relatively good health, and statistically my life expectancy is 84. A couple of years ago, I began to feel pressure (entirely self-imposed) to produce and accomplish more things. In lieu of a bucket list, I began to carefully weigh my priorities. I became more cognizant of my decisions. I knew that my choices mattered now more than ever. I banished certain activities I considered futile or non-essential, such as collecting CDs and wine. I stored my music digitally, stopped drinking alcohol, and sold my wine collection.

Aging reminds us that there is an opportunity cost to transactions. The upside is the ability to pursue things that truly inspire us — in my case, writing. I feel engaged and my mind is active when I write. With aging also comes the reality that I'm less mobile; fortunately, writing is a sedentary activity. Still, I am able to travel to see my children and grandchildren, including two trips to Hawaii each year (see essay 11). Family relationships top the bucket list for the majority of baby boomers.

In 2012, The Rolling Stones named their tour *50 & Counting*, which was not an exaggeration, considering "The World's Greatest Rock and Roll Band" is still going strong even after weathering the loss of drummer Charlie Watts. So, above all, I ask that the good Lord continues to "shine a light" on me. And now that I'm a half-decade past 64, I also ask that people still need me and feed me.

PROFESSIONAL DEVELOPMENT

∽

The First Time I Felt Like a Doctor

I was reborn as "Lazarus" when, as a resident, I went from feeling inadequate to becoming chief resident with new-found confidence. Sometimes it takes a breakthrough encounter with a patient or attending physician before you can relish your accomplishments.

THE TRUTH IS, I never felt like a doctor until I was in the final year of my residency. All through residency and medical school — and even before medical school — I wasn't sure I would ever really become a doctor. Heck, I barely got into medical school. I was accepted by only one program, and only on my second attempt. I spent my year off selling records at Sam Goody. And even they fired me!

I remember reading an article about doctors with MBA degrees — yes, I'm one of them — and the author made a distinction between business people with an MBA and doctors with an MBA. He said no one went to business school to become a doctor. In other words, even if MDs and DOs have postgraduate degrees, they wanted to become doctors first and foremost.

That was surely my case. I had wanted to be a doctor ever since I could remember. You could say my pediatrician made a good first impression. In kindergarten, the school's doctor (also a pediatrician) sent me home with a note after he conducted a routine physical exam. The note read: "Quite a normal boy."

"What did you say to him?" my mother wanted to know. I couldn't recall the exact conversation, but I remember discussing being overweight and that I loved meat and mashed potatoes. Laughter erupted from the nurse and doctor when I told them. I didn't understand why.

In my mind, I was destined to become a doctor. My aspiration to be a physician was always top of mind, until I attended a liberal college in Boston in the early 1970s. I became part of the "turn on, tune in, drop out" counterculture. Although I never met Dr. Timothy Leary, the Harvard psychologist who coined the infamous slogan, I did meet one of his contemporaries, B.F. Skinner, a pioneer of modern behaviorism, who wrote the book on operant conditioning and reinforcement theory.

In college, I became hooked on the study of behavior and switched my major from biology to psychology. I survived the cultural revolution, but, as I mentioned in the first essay, I graduated college with only a 3.4 GPA and subpar MCAT scores. My premed adviser said I would never get into medical school.

She was almost right. After a thorough trumping by a dozen or so schools, in which I was granted only two interviews (one of them obligatory from my alma mater), I had the chutzpah to call the other physician who interviewed me and showed a genuine interest in my application. Coincidentally, he was a psychiatrist, and he liked my essay, which was heavily tinged with references to mental health. It was fortuitous that we lived in the same city.

"Come to my house Saturday morning for coffee and we'll talk about it," he said over the phone. As a member of the admissions committee, any advice he could give me would obviously be welcomed. The psychiatrist told me to improve my GPA by taking a couple of science courses, study hard for the MCATs, and bring my science score up by 100 points (on a scale of 200 to 800). Wouldn't you know it, that's exactly what happened. (Thank you, Stanley Kaplan!)

The psychiatrist went to bat for me. "No need for a second interview," he said, offering to re-present my application to the admissions committee with improved scores. I was accepted into medical school. My dream had come true against all odds. Ironically, the psychiatrist and I would later become peers and clash over everything, from policy to treatment methods.

But here is where the story gets interesting. I trained at the same institution where I went to medical school (see essay 36). In my final year of residency, I was elected chief resident. As I recounted in essays 3 and 5, a patient attempted suicide while I was on call one evening, dealing a big shot to my ego. Although it wasn't my fault, I felt ashamed and blamed myself for the incident because I did not evaluate the patient (nor was I asked to) when I was consulted by phone by resident working in the emergency department. Self-doubt spiraled into anxiety and depression.

What kind of a doctor was I? One infatuated with medicine at an early age but barely accepted into medical school? An undergraduate psychology major with a disdain for science? A resident who let a patient slip through the cracks and almost die? A doctor with a business degree (yet to be earned)? I questioned my abilities and career choice.

My confidence booster finally came during my time as chief resident. I helped run the psychiatry department's consultation-liaison service, the arm of the department visible on the med-surg floors of the hospital. I was consulted about a patient who had attempted suicide by asphyxiation; he had put a plastic bag over his head to suffocate himself. His wife became alarmed, naturally, and the patient was admitted to the hospital by his doctor, a famous head-and-neck surgeon who also happened to be the father of one of my medical school classmates, as I highlighted in essay 9. Eight years earlier, the surgeon had explained to me and his daughter (my classmate) the detailed anatomy of the head and neck while helping us dissect a cadaver. I'm certain he didn't remember me this time, late on a Friday afternoon, when I was called to his patient's bedside.

After seeing the patient and his wife, I determined he was at high risk for suicide. The patient was reeling from a recent disfiguring operation for oral cancer, an operation that also left him literally and figuratively speechless. I suggested that the patient be transferred to the psychiatry unit for treatment of major depression. I didn't think he could wait to be seen as an outpatient.

The surgeon disagreed. "He'll be stigmatized," the surgeon told me. Our disagreement escalated into a toe-to-toe shouting match in the hospital corridor.

"He's already stigmatized," I exclaimed. "He's suffered enough." My reaction was swift and decisive. I didn't even pause to get the

OK for the transfer from the consultation-liaison attending. I did it reflexively, acting in the best interest of the patient.

My encounter with the surgeon turned out to be monumental. It signaled that I had arrived. In Eriksonian terms, years of shame and doubt gave way to autonomy, a latent breakthrough in my psycho-social development. For the first time in my life, I felt like a doctor.

Impact of Imposter Syndrome on Physicians' Practice and Leadership Development

Physicians with imposter syndrome have significant
difficulty suppressing feelings of inadequacy —
feelings that often persist throughout their career.

THE IMPOSTOR PHENOMENON (IP), also known as imposter syndrome (IS), was first described in 1978 by psychologists Pauline Rose Clance and Suzanne Imes. They defined it as an internal experience of intellectual phoniness in high-achieving women who seemed to be unable to internalize and accept their success. These women believed each new task would expose them as frauds, and they found countless ways to discredit their accomplishments despite receiving positive feedback and high accolades from their mentors and peers.

IS has since been observed in men and women in many high-stakes professions, including business, law, and medicine. Doctors who exhibit IS display symptoms common to other professionals such as anxiety, depression, shame, and burnout. In rare instances, suicide may result.

Symptoms of IS stem primarily from prolonged isolation and stress and an inability to meet self-imposed standards of achievement in individuals typically characterized as perfectionists and "type A" personalities, which encompasses most medical professionals. It is important to note, however, that IS does not necessarily equate with low self-esteem or a lack of self-confidence. The dominant theme is chronic self-doubt and a sense of intellectual fraud that overrides any feelings of success or evidence of competence.

Prevalence rates of IS in medical professionals vary widely, encompassing 22% to 60% or more of physicians and physicians in training. The pervasiveness was emphasized by a surgeon who commented, "I'd like to meet someone who HASN'T experienced imposter syndrome." In this vein, IS has been compared to burnout syndrome: Both constitute "a problem to be confronted at the organizational level with serious engagement from leadership and investment in both cultural transformation and policy change."

A 2016 study found that almost a quarter of male medical students and nearly half of female students experienced IS. Approximately one-third to one-half of medical residents have been identified as having IS. Even seasoned clinicians, those at advanced stages in their career, have questioned the validity of their achievements and reported feelings of imposture. Some believed they had "risen to the level of their incompetence," suggesting that past accolades could not buffer their insecurities, which they rarely shared with colleagues.

There is a robust literature that describes the negative association between IS and job satisfaction and performance leading to meaningful setbacks in the careers of some individuals and forcing others to abandon their profession altogether. Manifestations of IS that may adversely impact physicians and aspiring physician leaders include a lack of courage to take on new professional challenges, accept new assignments and projects, and learn new skills.

The symptoms of IS may be transient, but without treatment, IS is likely to be chronic with acute exacerbations of and anxiety and self-doubt when novel challenges and situations arise. It is not uncommon for IS symptoms to be present during medical training or when starting one's career, although some physicians may harbor life-long doubts about their abilities and believe it's only a matter of time before they're "found out."

Physicians plagued by IS, particularly those with misplaced self-doubt who are unable to accurately assess their skills and abilities and are unreceptive to corrective feedback, tend to become less motivated and less productive over time. They display self-handicapping behaviors such as procrastination and perfectionism. It's been said that perfection is the enemy of success, while a growth mindset is its greatest friend. Unfortunately, victims of IS are robbed of their growth potential.

Trainees and physicians with IS may feel unprepared for the next stage of their careers or future job prospects. They may avoid prominent leadership opportunities and fail to reach their full potential because the additional responsibility and visibility that comes with a leadership role intensifies their performance anxiety. In short, physicians with IS may be passed over for leadership positions, use flawed logic to exclude themselves from consideration, or fail as physician leaders.

A physician's feelings of phoniness can create a ripple effect. A physician's drive to pursue prestigious residencies, fellowships, or promotions may be thwarted by an inner voice that tells them they're not qualified and would not be selected. Doctors who believe they are imposters may behave in such a way as to cut short their potential to become physician leaders. IS could be the reason some promising physicians appear to have unfulfilled talent and are "held back" in their careers.

IS doesn't affect a person's ability to shoot, but it affects where they aim. This means that from a career perspective, despite significant achievements, physicians with imposter syndrome often aim low in order to limit their visibility lest others detect their (imagined) fraudulence. Their careers become truncated by mental paradigms that dictate "I am a failure," "I am a fake," and "I am not successful." In the mind of an imposter, success is the result of chance, and good luck will surely run out. Imposters pass up significant career opportunities because they are convinced they won't be able to do better elsewhere.

Recognizing that many trainees and newly minted physicians feel like imposters, my advice to them is as follows:

- Imposter syndrome is only a name. Don't let it derail you from your goals and aspirations.
- Realize that feelings of inadequacy are normal and ubiquitous among your peers. Don't be imprisoned by the fear of making mistakes — everybody makes them.

- Remember that the biggest misconception about Abraham Lincoln is that he was perfect. Cognitive distortions of your abilities and achievements are just that — distortions, which are correctable.
- You are not a fraud. You haven't gotten this far by accident. You have what it takes to be an excellent clinician and leader.

Chief Wellness Officer: New Opportunity, Necessary Role

Healthcare organizations are finally hiring physicians into the role of chief wellness officer to deal with alarming rates of burnout and mental health disorders in clinicians. The question is whether chief wellness officers will be swept aside in the C-suite — their titles perceived as gratuitous — or whether they will be given the necessary resources to effect real change.

NEARLY HALF THE PHYSICIAN WORKFORCE is considered unwell — burned out, depressed, in some cases suicidal. Unwell physicians provide suboptimal care to patients. Their patients' satisfaction scores are low. They are less productive than physicians who are well. They commit more medical errors, and their rate of malpractice litigation is higher. The work-life balance of a burned-out physician is way off-kilter — and tragically, about one physician per day dies by suicide in the United States.

All of these known effects have become attention-getting headlines. Healthcare organizations, however, have been slow to provide a fix despite the negative impact unwell physicians have on their bottom line — through staff turnover, lawsuits, decreased productivity, and disability claims. One meta-analysis showed that medical costs were lowered $3.27 for every dollar spent on wellness programs, and absentee day costs fell by about $2.73 for every dollar spent. The authors of the study concluded: "This return on investment suggests that the wider adoption of such [wellness] programs could prove beneficial for budgets and productivity as well as health outcomes."

Although other studies have failed to show financial returns on wellness programs, several high-profile institutions (e.g.,

Stanford, Johns Hopkins, Mount Sinai [New York], UC Davis, and the University of Alabama) have appointed chief wellness officers (CWOs) to counter staff burnout. They are discussing strategies and best practices in the cultivation of personal self-care and workplace wellness. They are beginning to allocate essential resources to help stem the tide of unhappy, dissatisfied, and impaired physicians. CWOs have been hired directly into the C-suite to work with other executives to deliver enterprise-wide solutions to drivers of burnout.

The essential responsibilities of the CWO vary by scope and type of organization. Based on my review of CWO positions described in academic healthcare systems, CWOs are tasked to establish a "Wellness" or "Work-Life" Center and manage the ongoing, day-to-day operations — clinical, business and budgetary — as well as oversee growth and expansion of the center. They are responsible for evaluating the center's impact on employee wellness, professional fulfillment, patient satisfaction, and patient safety. Ultimately, the CWO is responsible for creating and maintaining a system-wide culture of wellness by promoting and supporting staff well-being. This entails working with mental health leaders and department heads to decrease stigma and improve awareness and diagnosis of mental health disorders.

Of course, there are skeptics who believe that creating a CWO position simply satisfies an organizational checklist and pays lip service to the epidemic of burned-out doctors. It may create a distraction or deplete resources, they argue, unless the components of a physician wellness program are already in place: a wellness committee and leader, a burnout prevention strategy, a reasonable budget, up-and-running projects, and metrics to prove the program's effectiveness. The appropriate time to hire a CWO may be debatable, but one thing seems certain: Merely offering resiliency training under the guise of "wellness" puts the onus on physicians to deal with their own burnout and does not address its systemic causes.

The CWO will face several significant challenges: (1) establishing a working connection with front-line providers while based in the C-suite; (2) maintaining influence without being perceived as disruptive; (3) competing against other executive leaders for resources and status in the organization; (4) adding *immediate* value to the organization; and (5) demonstrating a return on investment for physicians (a highly specialized group for which the benefits of corporate wellness programs have been inconsistent).

But if the CWOs do their jobs effectively, senior leaders will forever be reminded of the importance of a culture that embraces psychological health and improves the professional lives of clinicians. Anything less jeopardizes the goals of the Triple Aim: improving the individual experience of care; improving the health of populations; and reducing the per-capita costs of care for populations.

Mental Health: The New "Coming Out" in Medicine

Individuals with mental disorders — and the clinicians treating them — have been stigmatized for centuries. Now with the recognition that the medical workforce is suffering higher rates of mental health problems than the general population, treatment is becoming more accepted. Openness about challenges with anxiety and depression can help fight the stigma.

SEVERAL DECADES AGO, it was inconceivable for physicians to admit they were gay, mainly because it was tantamount to career suicide. Sure, there were personal reasons to hide homosexuality — the stigma attached to gay and lesbian people was insufferable — but the medical establishment believed that homosexual doctors were mentally ill and not fit to practice medicine.

The term "homosexuality" was not fully removed from the Diagnostic and Statistical Manual of Mental Disorders until 1987. Until then, gay and lesbian doctors were denied residencies and university-based positions if their sexual orientation became known. Of course, a hiring bias against the LGBTQ+ community and other forms of discrimination remain today, but at the very least, these individuals are no longer considered mentally ill.

The same cannot be said of physicians who have openly admitted that they suffered from mental illness and who have written about their experiences. I applaud those physicians for sharing their stories and having the courage to "come out" and tackle mental health stigma head on. No one should be defined by a singular event in their life, whether it be a suicide attempt or psychiatric hospitalization, or by a lifetime struggle with depression or substance use. Once treated, unwell physicians provide the same quality of care as other physicians. I have been impressed with the accounts of recovered physicians and their efforts to shine a light on mental illness so that others can be led out of darkness.

Lately, I have seen a spate of self-reflections published in medical journals and on social media. I recount several of them here — published in June and July 2021 — to help raise awareness lest psychiatrically diagnosed doctors become shunned by the medical community as were their gay colleagues.

A Medical Student

A medical student wrote anonymously on *KevinMD* about their nearly two-decade struggle with depression, including several suicide attempts. The medical school administration shamed the student into silence and made no special provisions for help other than routine wellness initiatives. "Who do you talk to when your trusted advisers weaponize your mental illness as a weakness that should prevent you from becoming a doctor?" the student asked. Citing compelling statistics from one study — the prevalence of depression or depressive symptoms among medical students was 27.2% and that of suicidal ideation was 11.1% — the medical student offered several recommendations for medical schools:

- Designate a cadre of psychotherapists to treat medical students; ensure all therapists have diversity training to treat marginalized populations (i.e., black, indigenous, LGBTQ+, etc.).
- Separate the electronic medical record for mental health treatment from records of the hospital and medical school.
- Adopt a "help first" mentality and avoid punitive measures for students with mental illness.
- Educate the medical school faculty (and students) specifically about mental illnesses in students and provide relevant resources internal and external to the institution.

A Resident

In an essay published in *JAMA*, psychiatric resident Katherine A. Termini, MD, recalls how she deliberately overdosed at age 16 and, at the advice of her mentors, withheld her psychiatric history when she applied to medical school — her so-called "lie by omission." Termini continued her silence through medical school and residency interviews, fearing what a confession would do to her career, and also because clinicians made disparaging or dubious comments about suicidal patients.

She "came out" early in residency, no longer able to reconcile her shrouded past with her desire to become a psychiatrist and mental health advocate. Termini concludes: "Mental health stigma and the culture of self-sufficiency within medicine contribute to the continued suffering of physicians and trainees. Colleagues will continue to endure this injustice if this is not addressed on multiple fronts, from systemic changes to personal shifts in mentality and behavior."

A Physician

A story on Doximity was told by Mukund Gnanadesikan, MD, a psychiatrist, novelist, and poet. Gnanadesikan has experienced anxiety, depression, and suicidal ideation since college, although his worst suffering is far behind him. He readily shares aspects of his physical health with patients, but his psychiatric history is "one door [that] never opens...Who wants a doctor with a history of cerebral hiccups?" Gnanadesikan admits he has the same fear as his patients: the fear of being negatively judged for having a psychiatric history. Nevertheless, he believes his case is "proof that [mental] illness can be transcended, that those who consider themselves broken may one day heal others." A moving message no doubt, one that should instill hope in distressed physicians and inspire them to come forward.

What is my interest in this topic? I "came out" in 2014, nearly 30 years after I suffered emotional trauma related to a patient's suicide attempt — trauma that resulted in chronic anxiety and depression. I've written about my experience extensively in this book and elsewhere. Only by writing freely about mental health issues affecting the physician workforce can we encourage acceptance of mental illness among our patients and each other, and identify effective strategies for preventing and treating psychiatric disorders among physicians and those in training.

Are Your Hobbies Connected to Your Specialty?

*The issue of professional identity is complex, especially
for those of us who have significant interests outside of
medicine. Each activity informs the other, and being able
to fluidly go between them is a mark of flexibility that
can only enhance, not detract from, our roles as doctors.*

THROUGHOUT MY CAREER I have met doctors with some of the
most interesting hobbies: car collectors, wine makers, coffee roast-
ers, and many others. I've often wondered whether physicians who
have utilized their specialized skills in the practice of medicine have
parlayed those skills into hobbies. In other words, is there a connection between physicians' hobbies and their medical specialty? My
take is that doctors' hobbies and their specialty choices are often
inextricably linked.

To be sure, the COVID-19 pandemic drew considerable attention
to the importance of having a hobby. Physicians under prolonged
stress needed outside activities to decompress from hard-fought
battles lost and won on the COVID front lines.

According to a September 2020 U.S. Department of Labor report,
524,000 healthcare workers had left the field since February 2020,
doctors are among them. Of course, it's impossible to say whether
having a hobby would have mitigated the exodus, but the importance of having a hobby has been shown to be crucial in achieving
relaxation and work-life balance, as well as coping with anxiety,
depression, and traumatic medical experiences.

My son-in-law, for example, is a medical student and an avid
gardener. Gardening has allowed him to unwind from the pressure
of medical school while simultaneously parenting a newborn child.
Conversely, he feels that gardening has made him a better clinician
by teaching him to be patient, learning from failure, and accepting

death. Most importantly, gardening has taught my son-in-law concepts related to preventive medicine.

"Any gardener knows the importance of their soil's composition. You need to have the right amounts of organic matter, nutrients, minerals, fungi, and bacteria to give your plants the best foundation to grow. ... The garden has reminded me that in order to help our patients grow and maintain their health for longer periods of time, we must grant them solid ground beneath their feet and a clinician who can help them when needed," he wrote in an August 18, 2021 Doximity "Op-Med."

One of my most influential and admired professors (emeritus) at my medical school is infectious disease expert Bennett Lorber, MD, a professional painter. Lorber was raised in a family that valued art and music — his cousin is the accomplished jazz keyboardist and Grammy award-winner Jeff Lorber — and Lorber has painted since early childhood.

He also emphasizes the importance of having a hobby as a doctor. "Doing something that is important to you, makes you happy, and keeps you sane is just as important as what you do as a doctor. ... To best take care of patients, you have to first take care of yourself.... I am a doctor and a painter. Painting for me is not a hobby, but rather a calling equal to my calling to medicine," he says.

Some incredibly talented physicians have found their calling outside of medicine and have left the profession altogether. But the overwhelming majority are satisfied to straddle the fence, like psychiatrist and world-renowned jazz pianist Denny Zeitlin, MD, who maintains a private psychotherapy practice when not recording or touring.

On his website, Zeitlin discusses striking similarities between his two vocations: "The psychotherapeutic journey has commonalities with improvising music, which, as a jazz pianist and composer, has been another major passion. Empathy and communication are paramount in both, and I believe my most creative level of psychotherapy and musical expression occurs when I am able to trust that I will be able to bring to bear everything I have studied and learned while simultaneously allowing myself to be so immersed in the activity that I become 'one' with it — to merge with the music, the musicians, or the patient and his psychological life. I've been fascinated with the nature and challenges of this merger state. ... The cross-pollination of music and psychiatry has greatly aided me in both fields."

Success notwithstanding, Zeitlin is quick to add that his musical activities have always remained subordinate to his primary responsibilities to patients and trainees (he teaches at the University of California, San Francisco).

The same holds true for general surgeon and kiln-formed glass artist Steven Immerman, MD, who specializes in treatment for pilonidal disease. "Though I was extremely busy, I knew I needed a creative outlet," he says. "I found I really missed having a hobby in which I could use my hands. I was a surgeon at work, but even at play, I needed to work with my hands."

Once when Immerman attended a workshop and proposed a project — a block of colored glass with a window through which viewers could observe the contents inside — the instructor remarked, "Well, of course. You're a surgeon. You make little openings in people and you look inside."

Immerman has since observed similar parallels between people's choice of work and their extracurricular activities. Perhaps the most profound parallel can be seen in his own practice, because surgical and artistic outcomes both entail a period of waiting and uncertainty. "They both have a period of time when the process is seemingly out of my control," he says. "For surgery, it is the patient's healing process; for kiln-formed glass, it is the time it is in the kiln. Then, hopefully, there is the joy of seeing the finished product in both endeavors." Immerman also cited the example of a pathologist friend who enjoys astronomy in his spare time. "Both activities consist of looking through a lens and making order out of chaos," he observes.

I have searched for correlations in my own career, as an established psychiatrist and an amateur musician who collects rock and roll live music recordings. As best I can determine, with psychotherapy as my currency, the flow of the therapeutic conversation (the melody), combined with the spoken word of the patient (the lyrics), unites my practice with my hobby.

The relationship between work and hobbies need not be esoteric. For example, Christos Ballas, MD, a very busy ob/gyn, trains for and competes in triathlons. He notes, "My hobby is like my career, a big grind, but a lot healthier than going to work. I train and do endurance events, so when not working I'm swimming, running, or biking and thankful that at 61 I can still do it and practice full scope ob/gyn."

I invited physicians blogging on Doximity to share their views about the similarities between their hobbies and medical specialties. A plastic surgeon stated that he makes large-scale production model cars. "Maybe my hobby makes me a different kind of 'plastic' surgeon," he surmised. Emergency medicine physician and author Jeffrey Wade, MD, commented, "Stories are a way I receive the world as a big reader and how I report it back. Writing stories from my life has almost been like psychotherapy and gives me individual stories or books to hand out to people who seem like they could benefit from it" (also see the Afterword).

A retired ER trauma physician stated that he builds and shoots black powder Buffalo rifles from the 1800s and percussion muskets and flintlocks from the 1700s. What a curious hobby, I thought, for a physician who has probably treated hundreds, if not thousands, of gunshot victims during his career.

Physicians who are accomplished in their specialties and hobbies usually thrive on the interplay between them. It makes sense that our hobbies reveal a great deal about our passions and the activities that sustain us. Although our hobbies may not always align with our work, it's possible that the more they do, the higher our level of job satisfaction.

In fact, when graduating medical students were asked to rank the most important factors that influenced their specialty choice, "fit with personality, interests, and skills" consistently ranked the highest, behind specialty content, work-life balance, length of residency, and income expectations. The factors motivating physicians to pursue certain career pathways may be the very same factors leading them to choose lifelong hobbies.

Create a New Medical Reality

The process of career transition can be confusing. It doesn't have to be, however, if we consider ourselves free agents — essentially a "company of one," capable of defining our career pathways. Make sure you have your core competencies in tow, along with a knowledgeable and diverse "board of mentors."

TWO DOMINANT THEMES I'VE ENCOUNTERED among bloggers are embodied in the following headlines: "We must help physicians at the brink of burnout, depression, and high stress" and "Health care has crossed into a realm of moral injury and systemic collapse."

A physician responding to one of my op-eds inquired why the physician attrition rate in hospitals and clinics is so high. "What if there is no one left to stop the bleeding because we all have left the building?" he asked. I replied emphatically: "Get out of the spiral deathtrap now, while you can, relatively emotionally intact (I presume) before you become a statistic — either by suicide (God forbid) or as one of the 500,000+ healthcare workers who have left medicine since the onset of the pandemic."

Elvis may have left the building, but I bet many physicians will remain inside for a while. We are a highly resilient group, extremely dedicated, sometimes unfazed by the broken healthcare system. That's because some of us specialize in areas that have minimal interaction with the system's broken parts.

However, hospitalists, intensivists, ER docs, and PCPs are on the front line of care; their well-being will always be in question. I suggested that the aforementioned physician find a job with a better work-life balance, even if it meant subjugating his passion for medicine for a 9-to-5 job. After all, medicine is just a job — nothing more — run by the "suits" at the expense of doctors. Maybe the physician should seek employment in industry, e.g., pharma, health insurance or government. I encouraged him to speak out against his employer and attach his name to his opinions. The fear of retaliation should not silence good doctors (see essays 62 and 63).

I firmly believe that our choices within the medical profession are virtually unlimited. However, there is no more reason to stay in a job that is intolerable than it is to stay in a toxic relationship. Switch medical jobs before burnout and other forms of emotional exhaustion set in. Create a new reality rather than try and change the existing one.

My beliefs have deep roots in psychological experiments I read about in college. The first experiments were conducted by the physiologist Walter Cannon in the 1920s. He was the individual who described the fight-or-flight response. Cannon realized that a chain of rapidly occurring reactions inside the body helped to mobilize its resources to deal with threatening circumstances.

The term "fight-or-flight" represents the choices that our ancestors had when faced with danger in their environment. Many physicians facing this dangerous situation today, however, neither fight nor flee. They seem to be frozen at work, paralyzed by fear. They accept whatever comes down the pike, whatever the powers-that-be hand to them, like an obedient dog, which brings me to the second series of experiments.

The studies were conducted in the 1960s and 1970s by the psychologist Martin Seligman. He showed that dogs subjected to painful shocks made no attempts to avoid them when given the chance, e.g., by jumping over a barrier. Research on what is now known as "learned helplessness" has shown that when people feel like they have no control over what happens, they tend to simply give up and accept their fate. This maladaptive passivity is highly evident in physicians who feel trapped at work and see no future in practicing medicine. The condition of learned helplessness has become a model for major depression, and it can also explain burnout.

I was fortunate to have trained in an era when practicing medicine was not dominated by business concerns and electronic medical records and when most physicians worked autonomously and were self-employed. It seems we have crossed a chasm now — health systems employ the majority of physicians — and there is no changing the landscape, no going back. We protest, but because the medical profession is (and has been) engaged in an internecine war, there is no uniting force to change the present-day circumstances encumbering medical practice. We cannot declare *force majeure* for events that are foreseeable. This is the reality we are stuck with, and it is unlikely to improve.

But all is not hopeless. Here are two things to remember. First, Seligman became curious about why some individuals did not feel helpless even when hardened by their natural environment. He eventually focused his research on optimism and positive psychology. The aim of positive psychology is to begin to catalyze a change from a preoccupation with repairing the worst things in life to weathering them through optimistic thinking. There is no reason, Seligman believed, that people can't learn to be optimistic — an outlook we begin to cultivate by challenging and changing our automatic negative thoughts.

Second, I'd like to remind younger physicians who feel helpless and hopeless that even in my era, although practicing medicine may have been more enjoyable, many of my colleagues and I tried out different jobs to obtain the best fit (see essay 27). I actually spent half my career working in non-clinical positions. There were no chains on us then or now. I considered myself a free agent. I called my own shots. I worked on my own terms. When someone or some force changed those terms to my disliking, I went elsewhere, but I always landed a job in a medical-related field.

The guiding principle throughout my career has been to act as a "company of one" — advice given by Ronald N. Yeaple in his book *The Success Principle*. In other words, act as the CEO of your own career. In your "micro-corporation," your core competencies report to you, and you report to your board of mentors. That is the only reality that matters.

Discouraging Our Children from Becoming Doctors

I'm upset that so many physician parents have negative views about medical practice and are against medical careers for their children. They truly represent the "Great Resignation" in medicine.

BY NOW, MOST OF US ARE FAMILIAR with the term the "Great Resignation" — the tidal wave of people quitting their jobs in the United States and around the world. The Great Resignation began primarily in response to the coronavirus pandemic, but additional factors have sustained it.

Healthcare is the second largest sector hit by the Great Resignation (food services is number one). When questioned during the pandemic, one in five physicians and two in five nurses said they intend to leave their practice by the end of 2023. We used to say that healthcare costs are no longer sustainable. We can now drop the word "costs" and still be correct.

The term "Great Resignation" was coined by organizational psychologist Anthony Klotz, PhD, MBA, an associate professor of management at May Business School at Texas A&M University. Klotz explains, "From organizational research, we know that when human beings come into contact with death and illness in their lives, it causes them to take a step back and ask existential questions like what gives me purpose and happiness in life, and does that match up with how I'm spending my [time] right now? So, in many cases, those reflections will lead to life pivots."

Perhaps the most disturbing trend of the Great Resignation is the long-term implications. In order for resignations to be filled — especially doctors' jobs — we should be encouraging our children to consider a career in medicine, along with other, more immediate measures aimed at boosting staffing levels.

Stimulating an interest in the field of medicine is a good long-term strategy to replenish healthcare jobs. Not uncommonly, one or both parents who are — or were — physicians plant the seed to become a doctor early in their children's lives. The seedlings are cultivated with loving care until they germinate into premedical students, accepted into medical school on their own merit or as "legacy" students. In either case, some individuals would not have become doctors if it weren't for encouragement from their parents and high praise lavished upon the medical profession.

However, at a time when burnout and exhaustion are widespread, many physicians debate whether or not they would advise their children to follow in their footsteps. Even Hippocrates was uncertain about the rewards of a career in medicine. "The life so short, the craft so long to learn," he famously said. The crux of the matter is often viewed in terms of a tradeoff between the time invested to become a doctor and the return on investment — not only the financial return, but especially the personal gratification of practicing medicine.

A poll conducted by Doximity is quite revealing. Of approximately 12,000 physicians who responded to an online survey in January 2022, 60% said they would probably or definitely not want their children to work in medicine.

The most common reasons were those we've been reading about for the past decade: heavy caseloads, long hours, loss of autonomy, third party intrusions, and toxic workplace cultures. One family medicine physician asked: "Why make them [our children] suffer what we are suffering in this horrible situation created by EHRs, insurers, burocrats (sic), and so on and so forth?"

To be sure, a vocal minority did advocate for the profession. "I would be so proud to see my children continuing in this noble profession," a telemedicine physician commented. A neurosurgeon incredulously asked, "What can be more satisfying than saving lives?" A geriatrician said, "It's a great joy for me to see the likes of [my daughter] and her friends entering our still sacred profession and I hold out hope that they can smooth the rough edges."

That sentiment was echoed by many physicians who said that medicine was a worthwhile profession, calling it a "privilege," but only if their children have the "passion" and "desire" to enter practice. That makes me wonder, how much influence do we actually have over our children's career choices? While we cannot decide their future, we can encourage an interest in STEM and introduce them to the field of medicine through career fairs and job shadowing. But at the end of the day, most children will follow their hearts and not our wishes or dreams.

Three of my 4 adult children are healthcare practitioners. They made their own career decisions, and I encouraged and supported them. I didn't try to steer any of them into medicine, although I've always believed it was a great profession and told them so.

I'm afraid, however, that not enough physicians share my conviction. I'm saddened by surveys that indicate that nearly half of physicians would not choose medicine again. The moniker the "Great Resignation" can also be applied to those among us who hesitate to speak proudly of our profession and promote medicine as an honorable career — one worthy to serve the suffering, to paraphrase William Root, MD — and who fail to inspire promising students to choose medicine as a career.

The story I've repeatedly told my children (and others) comes from the "Field of Dreams," the scene where Ray Kinsella tries to persuade Dr. Archibald ("Moonlight") Graham to travel back in time to experience a once in a lifetime opportunity: a chance to bat in the major leagues. Dr. Graham refuses to go with Ray, and Ray exclaims: "It would kill some men to get so close to their dream and not touch it. God, they'd consider it a tragedy." To which Dr. Graham replies, "Son, if I'd only gotten to be a doctor for 5 minutes...now that would have been a tragedy."

Going Mobile – An Antidote for Career Regret

One of my favorite Who songs, "Going Mobile," inspired me to write about the virtues of switching jobs — even careers within medicine — to keep things fresh. Physicians have more capacity than they realize, and they have leverage to negotiate jobs that will sustain their interests over time.

In 2022, the National Resident Matching Program provided matching services to more than 42,000 applicants. A medical student's choice of specialty is one of the most important decisions they will ever make. But deciding which medical specialty to enter can be difficult. The majority of medical students are indecisive about their intended area of practice. Over the course of medical school, only a quarter (26.1%) of medical students who graduated in 2020 indicated the same specialty preference as they had when they began medical school.

Increasingly, U.S. medical students are choosing specialty and subspecialty practice rather than primary care, perhaps because certain specialties are constantly evolving and hold more interest than primary care practice. Boredom in a physician's specialty results in burnout and career choice regret. In fact, once in practice, nearly 1 in 5 physicians change their specialties to unrelated fields. Many others, however, feel trapped and unfulfilled.

The results of the 2022 Match speak to the attractiveness and strength of specialty practice compared with primary care practice. The most competitive specialties were emergency medicine, pediatrics, interventional radiology, otolaryngology, physical medicine and rehabilitation, diagnostic radiology, and various surgical subspecialties. On the other hand, the percentage of primary care positions filled by U.S. medical school seniors in 2022 declined 0.7% from 2021.

Career choice regret has been the focus of numerous researchers, and they have learned that the reasons for feeling regretful are a mixed bag of personal preferences, organizational fit, and unique characteristics of the work intrinsic to certain specialties. The truth is, physician regret is seen in all specialties as well as in primary care. It may be slightly higher in primary care because specialists are generally better compensated and their focus is usually restricted to a specific problem or patient complaint. In contrast, primary care physicians have a wider scope of practice. They must deal with many different problems, and not all physicians thrive on doing comprehensive exams for patients with multiple problems and comorbidities.

Yet, for some physicians, primary care has more versatility than specialty practice. Family medicine physicians, for example, can practice urgent care, traditional family medicine, women's health, pediatrics, integrative medicine, addiction medicine, or hospitalist and palliative care. So, in some ways, physicians who choose primary care practice may feel less regret because of the ability for family and internal medicine physicians to pivot.

Regardless, remorse over choosing a particular specialty is entirely different from remorse related to choosing medicine as a profession. Career choice regret addresses whether doctors would choose to become physicians again if they were able to revisit their career choices. According to a study published in *JAMA* in 2018, 14.1% (502) of 3,751 resident physicians said they would not choose to become doctors again. When it came to the choice of their actual specialty, 7.1% (253) indicated they would "definitely not" or "probably not" choose the same specialty if given another opportunity.

Could it be that staying in medicine, as opposed to switching specialties, is the more critical decision of the two? Perhaps physicians who are content with medicine as their chosen profession show the least amount of regret as long as they are able to traverse the system as their interests dictate. As discussed in essay 66, physicians have a multitude of options about how they work and on what terms they practice, in part because their core generalist education extends their reach and job flexibility.

I experienced regret during my residency — not for choosing to be a physician, but for choosing to be a practicing psychiatrist. I lost interest in seeing patients as my residency progressed, and by the time I was in academic practice, I knew it was time to bail and find another calling. My focus had changed from one-on-one patient care to population health. I changed jobs to work for a health insurance company in the newly emerging areas of quality assurance and utilization management. Eventually, I worked beyond the boundaries of mental health and supplemented my medical degree with a business degree (essay 71).

After working in the health insurance industry, I started a career in the pharmaceutical industry, working initially as a medical liaison and later in R&D and medical affairs. I had always had a strong interest in pharmacology and the neural mechanisms underlying behavior. And wouldn't you know it, the rave in psychiatry today is the repurposing of psychedelics as therapeutic agents to treat a wide variety of disorders including depression and PTSD.

You could say I went "mobile" to sustain my attraction to medicine and satisfy my whims, to explore all that medicine has to offer. My career is not a paradigm for overcoming career regret. Rather, it simply points out that job mobility may be an antidote for an initially wrong choice of a specialty and that leaving the medical profession may be an unnecessarily drastic move.

Medicine offers many fulfilling, meaningful, and lucrative opportunities to practice — or not. In addition to changing specialties, physicians are turning to combinations of "location-independent" jobs stacked with side jobs that additively lead to a preferred quality of life. Such is the nature of my work today.

If you have career remorse, think hard about the myriad opportunities within the medical field before calling it quits. Only then can you truly say you've left with no regrets.

Medical Leaders Must Show Their True Colors

If it's true that at some level all physicians have the capacity to lead, then they must show their true colors. Now is not the time to appoint physician leaders who only view the world through rose-colored glasses.

COLOR IS OFTEN USED AS A METAPHOR for personality and emotion. Terms like "red in the face," "feeling blue," and "green with envy" are etched in the vernacular. Great leadership requires emotional intelligence, and the best leaders lead in full color.

Colorful leadership is about seeing the whole picture, unfiltered by our own preferences and experiences. Colorful leaders have been depicted in books, movies, and songs. The "flower exercise" was at the heart of the number one best-seller *What Color Is Your Parachute?*, a book that culminates in a one-page What Color Is Your Parachute flower diagram of the reader's unique flower that provides a visual summary of their personality as it relates to their career development, goals, and objectives.

Cyndi Lauper's smash hit "True Colors" is about looking below the surface to see what a person is really like. The song is about being unafraid to show your true colors — in other words, to be yourself. "True Colors" took on special meaning in the gay community, which is represented by a rainbow pride flag. (Lauper has long been a supporter of LGBTQ+ rights.)

I came across a compilation of songs by the French jazz pianist Michel Petrucciani (1962–1999). The compact disc (CD) is titled "Colors." The CD cover displays the colors of the rainbow in the shape of a record album and 10 qualities representative of Petrucciani's music. The same qualities, in my opinion, can be found in the best medical leaders. Briefly, they are:

1. **Action.** Medical leaders are action-oriented. Their goals are achieved by doing rather than dictating. Medical leaders serve as an example and role models for others.

2. **Dignity.** Medical leaders treat everyone with kindness, compassion, and respect. They embrace diversity and inclusiveness in the workforce.

3. **Spiritual.** Emerging research has shown that healthcare leaders who are more developed in terms of their spirituality are highly effective leaders and achieve more positive results for their organizations. Spiritual leaders have been shown to reduce burnout among healthcare workers.

4. **Sentimental.** Patients possess strong sentiments about the healthcare they receive. Virtually every interaction with a provider or hospital will trigger a positive or negative reaction, immortalized in online reviews. As a result, sentimental leaders are extremely valuable to their organizations. They are empowered to optimize the patient experience and enhance business outcomes on a larger scale.

5. **Serious.** Promoting individuals for leadership and management roles is a serious concern with global implications. It requires a deep commitment to aspiring leaders as well as policymakers who must have the courage to give autonomy to and support medical leaders.

6. **Passive.** Passivity is usually cited as a reason leaders fail, and there is no doubt that inertia in task completion is a major problem for some physicians. But for the majority who are action-oriented, when it comes to their personal lives, medical leaders need to learn how to offset their frenzied work schedules and take care of themselves. Some leaders find the entire concept of self-care to be antithetical to their image of a great leader who is perceived as always on the go. News flash: Leaders need self-care, too!

7. **Peaceful.** Peacebuilding in the medical profession is critical. It has been suggested that medical leaders have the ability to contribute to peacebuilding efforts worldwide by analyzing and resolving conflict and building trust among people and

organizations. As opposed to the many toxic characteristics that have come to dominate leadership circles in the United States, experience from the United Kingdom shows that a peaceful and level-headed approach to managing medical systems correlates with better quality of care, better financial performance, higher levels of patient satisfaction, lower levels of staff stress and, in hospitals, a lower level of avoidable patient mortality in organizations.

8. **Violence.** Violence is an odd descriptor to associate with Petrucciani's music, given that the music is highly lyrical. Yet, violence and medicine are not strange bedfellows. Violent encounters between patients and medical personnel are all too common. Furthermore, medical errors have been responsible for perpetuating violence, albeit unintentionally, against the very individuals medical practice intends to help. More than ever, healthcare leaders must focus on reducing medical error and detecting burned-out and impaired physicians who unwittingly cause harm to their patients.

9. **Sorrow.** Medical leaders must understand and deal with long-term periodic sadness that the chronically ill and their caregivers experience in reaction to continual losses. They must learn to support their grieving colleagues and know when normal grief reactions have morphed into pathological forms of grief, such as clinical depression. This is especially difficult in light of the controversy, both within and outside the field of psychiatry, regarding the boundaries of normal sadness and major depression.

10. **Happiness.** Cultivating happiness in medicine has become a key strategic objective of many graduate medical education programs. As discussed in essay 16, many institutions have appointed chief wellness officers to leadership roles and tasked them to implement and oversee a holistic and comprehensive plan to reduce burnout and bolster individual wellness.

Michel Petrucciani died from complications of osteogenesis imperfecta. Despite his physical limitations, chronic pain, and small stature — just 3 feet — he was a jazz piano giant. In his brief 36 years, Petrucciani recorded or appeared on more than 40 albums, many with jazz luminaries. He was the subject of several tributes and awards. Petrucciani was buried at Le Pere Lachaise Cemetery in Paris, one grave away from Frederic Chopin.

I wish the qualities embodied in Petrucciani's music were universal among medical leaders because right now, it seems they are viewing the world through rose-colored glasses.

I May Be Old School, but I'm Not Outdated

What is an "old school" physician? One individual commented: "This 'old school' 53-year-old psychiatrist…still does paper charts, sees follow ups for 30 minutes, runs on time, calls all her own patients back, and emails/calls therapists and internists who co-treat patients." Old school physicians are diligent, caring and patient-centric. They are unfettered from assembly-line medicine. They continually learn. They transcend generations, and they are anything but outdated.

I was not content to retire at age 65 like many of my contemporaries, some who exited medicine at an even earlier age. However, when I turned the golden age, my job was eliminated, as discussed in the preface. The problem I faced was not that I was suddenly retired; rather, it was that I hadn't retired into anything.

Left jobless, I thought long and hard about my next move. My only prerequisites were that whatever new work I undertook, it had to be portable so I could travel and visit my grandchildren who were scattered from the east coast to Hawaii. My "encore career" had to be location-independent (essay 21) and not involve direct patient care, not even via telehealth. I found that job in the form of a collaborating physician — a physician who supervises advanced practice providers (APPs: nurse practitioners or physician assistants).

The responsibilities of collaborating physicians vary from state to state and usually involve chart review at a minimum. I suppose reviewing the charts of APPs is considered a good proxy for evaluating their quality. However, I insist that in addition to reviewing charts, I talk directly with APPs and discuss their patients — similar to conducting "curbside consultations." These talks are quick and easy and give me a much better sense of the qualifications and expertise of the provider.

"Oh, Dr. Lazarus, you're so old school," I've been told.

What does it mean to be "old school?" A baby boomer? Educated before the proliferation of computers and PowerPoint? Attended classes in person rather than virtually? Charted hand-written notes before the advent of electronic medical records? Looked at patients rather than computer screens? Listened to their stories? Probably all the above and more.

Suneel Dhand, MD, an internal medicine physician and health and lifestyle coach, describes seven fundamental traits of old school physicians: attentive, not rushed, thoughtful, clinically astute, personally connected, independent, and technologically unchained. I believe old school values still appeal in modern medicine; patients and families seem to desire these qualities in physicians. In addition, strong physician-patient relationships promote better outcomes.

I'm proud to be an old school physician, even if the term "old school" carries a negative connotation. Thomas Cohn, MD, is a physiatrist and pain specialist who touts on his website the benefits of being old school. He notes that in many cases, old school medicine affords him the time to do a detailed history and physical examination and correlate signs and symptoms without the need for extensive laboratory and imaging studies.

Dhand states, "The old school physician has the diagnosis in mind right after talking to and examining their patient." That explains why I insist on personally supervising APPs — I'm more interested in how they treat their patients than how they treat their charts. Given that about half of the total text in the medical record is duplicated from text previously written about the patient, chart review is a waste of my time. Duplication also makes me doubt the veracity of the information in the medical record (essay 68).

The essence of my interactions with APPs is making sure they have captured the chief complaint, taken a full history (±physical exam for psych patients) including family and social history, and conducted a thorough review of systems and a mental status examination. I want to hear about the diagnosis, differential diagnosis, treatment plan, and response to therapy. You know, old school.

Every generation seems to consider the previous one "old school." The classic textbook *The True Physician: The Modern "Doctor of the Old School"* was written for young doctors by the scholarly physician Wingate M. Johnson, MD. The textbook contained "worldly wisdom," according to a review of the book in *JAMA*. Here's a revelation: The book was published in 1936, when Johnson was around 50 years old. The "young physicians" were probably half his age. Old school doctoring has been around a long time, always marked by generational gaps.

During medical school, some of my classmates ridiculed a senior attending physician whom they considered old school. He wore a bow tie, mumbled and fumbled his way through the hospital corridors, and always seemed to be in a hurry. The attending ran a busy outpatient practice in internal medicine, made house calls, and rounded on his hospitalized patients. Medical students considered him a dinosaur.

But the attending also instructed us in medical school and conducted clinical research, fulfilling the academic tripartite mission of clinician, teacher, and researcher. "Where does he get the time and energy to do all this?" students wondered. When Dhand encountered an old school physician, he asked a more incisive question: "How have we got to the stage where a genuine and caring doctor has become the odd one out?"

I think I know the answer.

The attending remained steadfast to his patients. They loved him and stuck with him for decades. The attending was versatile and efficient. Contrary to the stereotype of the old school physician who has let their knowledge lapse and lost their clinical skills, this attending was brilliant. In fact, he was the director of our medical school's continuing education department.

It was my supposition that the medical students feared they would not measure up to the attending once they became practitioners themselves, so they felt compelled to put him down. They mocked him by joking that every one of his chart entries read the same — "as above, see below" — in reference to the attending's heavy reliance on the house staff for the overall management of his patients. Rather than view the attending as a role model, they maligned and marginalized him for his seemingly old school ways. Yet, there was nothing about his thinking that was out of step with the times.

The use of "old school" as a pejorative term has its origins in ageism, as I discussed in essay 12. Labeling a physician "old school" compensates for trainees' insecurities and feelings of inadequacy. It's a riff from an old theme so eloquently explicated in *The House of God*: the desire for connection foiled by ageist (and other) assumptions that drive people apart. Sharing memes poking fun at the elderly only deepens divides.

While visiting my daughter, I related a story about someone close to us who got lost driving to the supermarket. When I tried to give this person the correct directions after the mishap, they got angry at me. "You were mansplaining," my daughter explained. To her surprise, I knew at once what the term meant, and I responded, "I may be old school, but I'm not outdated."

The Jobs You Hold Prior to Medical School Are Important, but Not for the Reason You Think

Medical school admission committees rely heavily on past experience working in the health field as a criterion for selection into medical school. I think it's more important to work at jobs that build character. "Cold beer" anyone?

MOST EXPERTS RECOMMEND that premed students seek medicine-related jobs to gain early proficiency and support their medical school application. There is nothing like valuable hands-on experience, they say, for students to demonstrate their passion and knowledge about the field of medicine. According to the article "25 Health Care Jobs To Get Before Medical School," written by the Indeed Editorial Team, "students who fill their resumes with volunteer work, research projects, and relevant work experience stand out as committed, stronger candidates within the medical field."

There are physicians who would disagree with Indeed. One of them is Stephen Klasko, MD, MBA, a healthcare "futurist" and obstetrician/gynecologist by training. Klasko led three different medical colleges and health systems before moving into consulting. In his book *Feelin' Alright: How the Message in the Music Can Make Healthcare Healthier*, Klasko remarks, "Everything I have learned personally and professionally … I owe to and can trace back to lessons I learned from being a DJ" — namely, self-awareness and the importance of understanding and listening to your audience. Here's the kicker: Klasko and I were high school classmates vying for air time as DJs at the student-run radio station.

Patrick Connolly, MD, MBA, a neurosurgeon practicing in Philadelphia, Pennsylvania, also disagrees with the Indeed Editorial Team. Before medical school, Connolly worked at a restaurant where he learned how to set tables, prioritize tasks, cater to diners' needs, and even make béarnaise sauce. Connolly learned the importance of teamwork, considered fundamental to the practice of medicine. Working in a restaurant instilled foundational skills and enabled him to discover the pleasure of serving others. A seemingly menial job before medical school prepared Connolly for a demanding career in neurosurgery. (His editorial appeared in the *Philadelphia Inquirer*, November 29, 2022.)

While reading Dr. Connolly's story, I had a flashback to the many mundane summer jobs I held in high school and college: stock boy at a women's shoe store, jack-of-all-trades at a textile factory, and beer vendor at a major league baseball park. The beer vendor job, in particular, is etched in my mind. I had a captive audience on the upper deck; the fans were always thirsty for a cold beer on a hot summer night. The profits from selling beer were second only to hawking hot dogs.

I was able to convince the manager of the food concession that I was of legal age (21) to sell alcohol. I was only 19 years old, but I was never asked to produce identification. Did I feel guilty? Heck, yes. Did I worry about getting caught? Sometimes. But nobody paid much attention to the vendors, especially those working in the "nose-bleed" section of the stadium. We were viewed as misfits and social outcasts, arriving early at the stadium to gamble our previous nights' wages at poker.

Vending at night games was a second or third job for some individuals. They were struggling to get by. "I'll never be like them," I thought. They would never amount to anything, and certainly, there were no doctors or potential doctors among them. I was dead wrong. My best friend, with whom I shared rides to the ballpark and was himself a hot dog vendor, became a family medicine physician.

My superior attitude no doubt was a reaction to my own insecurity about being able to "cut it" as a premed student, as well as my fear that I would be viewed in the same light as the derelict characters collectively referred to as "vendors." Most of all, I was embarrassed to be seen with them and indignant over the nature of the job.

One night, I encountered a high school classmate who was attending the game with her boyfriend. I sheepishly offered an explanation that I was working my way through college, hoping to get into medical school. Meanwhile, my classmate was already beginning to taste success as a fashion designer and was merely two years removed from high school.

I never discussed my job as a beer vendor with anyone who had anything to do with medical school. I omitted the experience from my medical school application, focusing instead on college "distinction" work at a Harvard-affiliated children's hospital. However, my ballpark experience came up during a "meet and greet" with the dean of my medical school. I was astonished when he included it in my "Dean's Letter" as part of my application to residency programs. I asked him to remove it, but he refused.

The dean stated, "Your job as a beer vendor shows you have character and adds color to your personality" (as if he had read essay 22). I thought peddling beer in front of half-stoned bleacher bums indicated *I* was a character. Who would want a buffoon for a resident shouting, "Cold beer!" and "Last call for alcohol!" ? I was afraid of being typecast as a loser.

The dean did not share my perspective. "Not a loser," he said, "a hard worker." He believed the ability to interact peaceably with rowdy fans was a strength that would serve me well in psychiatry, dutifully noting his opinion in my letter. Still, I never shared with the dean that I had lied about my age to get the job.

Quality guru Donald Berwick, MD, described a similar story in *JAMA*. He was a medical student interviewing at Peter Bent Brigham Hospital for a residency position. The day before the interview, his resident supplied him with the answer to a difficult question usually asked of prospective residents. Berwick chose to answer the question rather than confess he had been prepped for it by his resident. He aced the interview, but guilt set in shortly afterward, and Berwick dropped Brigham from his match list.

Berwick commented, "A choice came, on little cat feet, and I did not see it at the time for what it was. This is the moral choice in its simplest, purest, most elemental form. To tell the truth, or not, when 'not' is perhaps in your short-term self-interest." Lying was definitely in my short-term interest — not only to lie, but when the manager asked my age, I looked him squarely in the eye and said, "I'm 22," inflating my age by three years and going one beyond the legal age.

The dean was unaware I had a hidden agenda when I asked him to delete the job from his letter. My personal shame was not that I was a beer vendor; rather, I had told a bold lie to get the job. I'm not proud of it, yet from my reading, I discovered there are times when lying on behalf of patients may benefit them. And, if you believe Pamela Wible, MD, one of America's foremost physician advisors and advocates, doctors are actually trained to lie (see essay 51).

I emailed Connolly to congratulate him on his essay. He replied, "The stuff we do before we become other people shapes us in so many ways." I would add that "the stuff we do" goes well beyond the job itself. Early career jobs unrelated to medicine help shape our moral fiber and set our moral compass. "Ethics cannot be taken for granted," Berwick concluded.

When Being a Physician Leads to PTSD

As physicians, we are susceptible to PTSD because we have not been taught a healthy approach to being imperfect. Keeping everything bottled up and soldiering on has been acknowledged to be an inferior strategy to dealing with trauma. Institutions perpetuate trauma or look the other way on harm done to those who depend on them. When will the medical profession wake up and do the obvious work to care for its own practitioners proactively and effectively?

WHEN IT COMES TO TRAUMA, the focus of attention is our patients, recognizing their adverse childhood experiences and learning how to provide trauma-informed care. But what about us — the healers, the first responders, the listeners, the front-line physicians? Can practicing medicine also be considered a traumatic experience and risk factor for PTSD? If you've read a few of the essays in Section I, then you know the answer is "yes."

The concept of trauma as it relates to PTSD and early versions of the DSM depicts devastating events such as natural disasters, sexual assault, military combat, and physical attack. Over time, however, the DSM has expanded the list of potential stressors. Now, in its fifth, text-revised edition (DSM-5-TR), the manual recognizes indirect exposure to trauma, including aversive details of traumatic events, as possible stressors resulting in PTSD.

The DSM also states that professionals may be indirectly affected by trauma in their line of work — for example, psychotherapists exposed to details of their patients' traumatic events. However, the DSM does not identify physicians as indirect victims of trauma, even though they, like psychotherapists, may be exposed to traumatic events incurred by their patients.

The terms "secondary trauma" and "vicarious trauma" were introduced in essay 3. These terms have been used to define a spectrum of symptoms and conditions that have resulted from exposure to traumatic material or the account of patients' traumatic exposures during treatment. Vicarious trauma should be distinguished from trauma typically seen in PTSD — trauma that involves direct exposure to actual or threatened death, serious injury, or sexual and other bodily violence.

I became interested in vicarious traumatization toward the end of my first year of residency, when I was involved in an incident surrounding a patient's suicide attempt (see essays 5 and 17). Although the patient survived, I struggled to keep my emotions in check. I guess I failed, because many of the faculty noticed I had become anxious and depressed. I tried to "cherry-pick" my patients, avoiding, of course, those with suicidal ideation and other anxiety-provoking conditions. "What's wrong with Art?" my colleagues wanted to know. I was actually put on probation because my depression was affecting the quality of my work.

I reached out to a senior psychiatrist who helped me in therapy. My depression gradually lifted, and the whole ordeal was apparently forgotten by the time I was in my final year of residency. I was even appointed chief resident. But the scars of the trauma never completely healed. It was one of the reasons I began to transition to industry just seven years after my residency — to work in less stressful environments.

Since then, I have been researching the effects of vicarious trauma on those of us in healthcare. The extant literature indicates that PTSD occurs in 10–20% of physicians. Main stressors include treating trauma patients; working in conflict zones; working in underserved, remote, or rural areas; and the cumulative effects of on-the-job stress.

The incidence of PTSD in medical students and residents approximates that seen in practicing physicians, but the stressors tend to be different. Clinical situations that trainees might find traumatic include — but are not limited to — treating patients with mutilating injuries from high-speed motor vehicle accidents, falls, or burns; assessing and treating battered infants; assisting at an unsuccessful cardiac arrest, especially in a young or previously healthy patient; and being "pimped" and feeling put down, bullied, or humiliated by an attending physician.

PTSD symptoms in physicians increased during the COVID-19 pandemic, and the pandemic, itself, was declared a traumatic stressor. Although the threshold for full-blown PTSD may not have been met in all instances, healthcare workers experienced alarming levels of moral distress and moral injury during the pandemic — wounds from having done something, or failed to stop something, that violated their moral code. There is an evolving understanding that moral injury may set the stage for PTSD, often compounded by shame and guilt. Moral injury at the height of the coronavirus pandemic stemmed from being unable to provide adequate care to dying patients and counsel individuals on ways to slow the spread of COVID-19.

Physicians with PTSD have been compared to wounded soldiers insofar as the concept of moral injury was first described in service members who returned from the Vietnam War with symptoms that resembled PTSD. Though the trenches today's physicians are working in are non-literal, physicians may nevertheless suffer ongoing emotional trauma that may affect not only them, but also their families and patients. If not addressed promptly and appropriately, the emotional impact of trauma may influence a physician's career trajectory, as it did mine.

I have no regret about leaving practice, but other physicians I've spoken to have expressed remorse that they could not continue seeing patients due to PTSD. One physician wrote to me that he was traumatized by a malpractice lawsuit and further traumatized when pressured to settle out of court. Failing to "get his day in court," where he was certain he would be vindicated, largely contributed to his PTSD and "emotional inability to stay in practice." In fact, pushed to their limits by various stressors, one in five physicians intends to leave practice by 2024.

To counteract the Great Resignation described in essay 20, a three-tiered model to provide escalating support for physicians with PTSD has been recommended:

- Tier 1: Emotional support from trained peers (not "wounded" clinicians).
- Tier 2: One-on-one support and group debriefings when the whole team experiences an unexpected patient outcome.
- Tier 3: Referral to a professional mental health counselor specializing in PTSD and other trauma- and stressor-related disorders.

As clinicians, we have been tasked to learn and apply the principles of trauma-informed care to our patients to achieve better outcomes. A deeper understanding of the causes of trauma-based disorders and their treatment also opens our eyes to issues we may have overlooked or ignored in ourselves — namely, the toll of medical practice on our psyche and well-being.

Trauma Motivated Me to Become a Doctor

The preceding essay reviewed how practicing medicine may cause PTSD. But the opposite is also true: Personal trauma may motivate some individuals to enter the medical profession in order to help themselves and others.

"RAISE YOUR HAND if you told the person who interviewed you for medical school that you wanted to become a doctor to help people. I see practically every hand in the room raised. Keep them raised if you told your interviewer you also wanted to become a doctor to overcome personal trauma."

Everyone lowered their hands.

"I'm dismayed there are no honest people here," I joked to attendees at an annual meeting of the American Psychiatric Association (APA), where two colleagues and I conducted a workshop on "PTSD in Physicians."

And so, I launched into my presentation to the standing-room-only crowd. Most of the attendees were psychiatrists. As discussed in the previous essay, psychiatrists suffer a relatively high rate of PTSD because they are exposed to aversive details of their patients' traumatic experiences, not unlike first responders exposed to serious injury or death. Emergency medicine physicians and rural primary care physicians also have higher rates of PTSD compared with the general population.

Also, as I discussed in earlier essays, indirect exposure to trauma, also called vicarious or secondary traumatization, has long been overlooked by the medical profession as a possible cause of PTSD. However, according to a 2011 study published in the *Archives of Surgery*, nearly 80% of residents and physicians said they faced either an adverse event or a traumatic personal event in the preceding year. Whereas the lifetime prevalence of PTSD among adults in the United States is approximately 7% , it's roughly twice that percentage for medical students, residents, and practicing physicians.

Previously, only individuals who suffered direct trauma (e.g., physical attacks, natural disasters, severe motor vehicle accidents) were considered candidates for a diagnosis of PTSD. But following changes in the DSM-5-TR in conjunction with health threats associated with the coronavirus pandemic and the recent increase in mass shootings and killings in the United States, including watching violent media coverage, the incidence of vicarious trauma appears to be on the rise.

When I asked the workshop participants for a show of hands, it was unclear whether the type of trauma they might have considered was primary or secondary. I suspect both were in play, if for no other reason than I have personally experienced the effects of direct and indirect trauma. I also pushed toward medicine — psychiatry, in particular — hoping I would learn how to deal with the trauma I suffered during childhood and adolescence.

Many aspiring medical students admit to being attracted to medicine because of personal, medical-related experiences such as a serious illness in themselves or a family member. I imagine that personal trauma is also a factor, although few admit it, as witnessed in the workshop.

I conducted an internet search of "trauma as a motivation factor to become a doctor" and came up empty. Yet, medical school applications are replete with students' accounts of surviving cancer and other near-death experiences. Perhaps the students don't see it as trauma and instead justify their reasons for wanting to become a physician (apart from "helping others") as "improving the quality of life" and "taking steps toward disease prevention."

During my formative years, I endured the type of trauma that leaves a permanent scar on your psyche, takes away your confidence, and robs you of an identity. I'm talking about teasing, bullying, and peer rejection. It was nothing as serious as cancer or a life-threatening event, but it was life-changing.

Adverse childhood experiences are strongly correlated with PTSD. My first memory in life occurred when I was approximately six months old. It was traumatic. I remember being in an "old age" home with funky smells. My parents handed me off to my immigrant grandparents. I did not want to be with them. I immediately began crying. I found solace only when I was returned to the comforting outstretched arms of my mother.

Shortly afterward, at home, with my mother away and my father at work, our housekeeper put me in my crib for an afternoon nap. I wasn't tired. I did not want to sleep. I began crying. The housekeeper slammed the door to my room. I cried myself asleep.

I guarantee these are not false memories, nor is it impossible to remember events as early as the first year of life. Many have a lingering effect. Although my experiences were traumatic, they were not unique. We all suffer psychologically damaging incidents growing up — some of us more than others — and we tend to keep them hidden. How many of us aspire to become doctors partly because, consciously or not, we seek to be healed of our trauma or learn how to render first-aid to ourselves?

When you add the trauma from our childhood plus the secondary trauma from practicing medicine, do we not see ourselves as wounded warriors? As physicians, we are considered worthy to serve the suffering, but are we not worthy of salvation? Any physician who has not yet dealt with trauma should run — not walk — to a trauma specialist and seek their help and guidance.

At the APA workshop, a young psychiatrist bravely shared a personal account. She had been working at a VA hospital for several years and was currently going through a divorce. She felt traumatized by what was happening at work and in her personal life. She was most upset about treating veterans and listening to the unimaginable horrors of combat. She broke down and started to cry as she related her story.

I have periodically kept in touch with this psychiatrist. I am happy to report she entered therapy, left her husband, and left practice for a nonclinical career. She is doing well.

However, a substantial proportion of patients who seek treatment for PTSD continue to remain symptomatic, with impaired levels of functioning. This lack of progress in PTSD treatment has been labeled as a national crisis, calling for an urgent need to find a more effective therapy. The first step, however, is recognizing that, as healers, we are highly vulnerable to trauma, beginning early in life and continuing throughout our practice years.

Avoid Burnout by Finding Your Fit in the Organization

Burnout can be an outgrowth of a persistent culture clash at work. It causes high levels of job dissatisfaction and disengagement. Physicians who recognize the importance of cultural fit and attain it are more likely to be happy and productive.

STUDIES HAVE SHOWN a national burnout rate of more than 50% among physicians in practice. A 2018 survey conducted by Merritt-Hawkins revealed 78% of physicians sometimes, often, or always experience feelings of burnout. Physicians who transitioned from independent practice to employment in healthcare organizations reported higher rates of burnout, suggesting that working for large integrated health systems may not be an antidote for private practice-related stress.

As physicians seek employment, they should consider the "goodness of fit" between themselves and the organization. In the field of statistics, *goodness of fit* describes how well a model correlates with actual observations or values. Organizational psychologists borrowed the term to describe the compatibility of a person's temperament and skills with workplace requirements and environment. (Goodness of fit should not be confused with fitness for duty, which determines whether an individual can safely perform a defined job.)

The interaction between workplace variables and physician characteristics profoundly influences the effects of work. The ultimate consequence of a poor fit is disillusionment, pessimism, burnout, and depression. Although major depressive disorder and burnout are clinically distinct entities, there is significant overlap in symptoms.

The cardinal manifestations of burnout syndrome — exhaustion, cynicism, and reduced personal accomplishment — threaten the health and well-being of physicians and, by extension, their patients. It is important for physicians to examine the goodness of fit prior to accepting a job offer in an organization lest they become victims of overwhelming work demands, prolonged stress, and other causes of burnout.

The impact that work has on an individual's mental health and well-being is undeniable. It is said that at the height of his prominence nearly 100 years ago, Sigmund Freud was asked, "What is life all about?" He responded with two words: "liebe und arbeit" (love and work). ("Play" was added years later.) Mental health benefits accrue when work is characterized by certain features common to good-fitting jobs.

Research has shown that individuals who fit in well with their organizations report higher levels of job commitment and satisfaction and less anxiety, depression, and substance use. In addition, working for a good-fitting organization leads to high individual productivity, low absenteeism, and few disability claims.

Although no single set of job characteristics is good or bad for everyone, and although job requirements may change over time, research indicates 10 conditions are important, perhaps prerequisite, for a good fit between physicians and organizations, and may diminish professional burnout:

1. **Type of Organization.** Organizations involved in mergers, acquisitions, downsizing, outsourcing, and other economic forces beyond their control put physicians' job security at risk. Continued exposure to market dynamics over which they have no control threatens physicians' job security and may lead to physician burnout.

2. **Reporting Relationships.** Persistent conflict with a supervisor, a board member, or a key stakeholder can shorten the tenure of employed physicians. New bosses who may be intent on replacing their direct reports with friends and former colleagues in a proverbial housecleaning may be difficult supervisors. Frontline leaders with poor leadership qualities have negative effects on the personal well-being and job

satisfaction of the physicians they lead and burn them out over time.

3. **C-Suite Climate.** Physicians seeking employment as executives should gauge the temperament of non-physician executives with whom they will be working. Dissimilarities between physician executives and other leaders in the C-suite are the result of distinctive and different processes of training and professional socialization, as well as differences in psychological makeup.

4. **Communication.** Joseph Grenny, author of *Crucial Conversations* and "Speak Up or Burn Out," observes that physicians who engage more consistently and effectively in conversations that strengthen their social support systems and give them a greater sense of efficacy are less likely to burn out. Crucial conversations also breed powerful organizations toward which physicians gravitate.

5. **Career Development.** Physicians often cite stalled careers and lack of opportunity for advancement as reasons for burnout. Low morale and burnout often set in when physicians are not allowed to explore alternatives to traditional medical practice or are denied capital and other resources to remain competitive and cutting edge in their specialty.

6. **Clear and Unambiguous Roles.** Studies have shown that role conflict and role ambiguity are significant factors in work stress among employees. When a clear path is not in sight, it is only natural for organizations to flounder and eventually fail for lack of focus and direction. Practicing under these conditions deflates physicians' morale and contributes to burnout.

7. **Goal Alignment.** Organizations and physicians need alignment of goals to create safe and high-quality care at lower cost (see essay 6). Mutually rewarding goals lead not only to business success, but also personal satisfaction. Goals that resonate with one's sense of purpose and meaning are likely to appeal to physicians, as are personal challenges and projects that lead to highly valued outcomes.

8. **Rewards and Retention.** Formalized physician reward and retention programs are growing in popularity. Rewards provide a competitive advantage in recruitment and help create camaraderie among the medical staff that is essential to preventing burnout. Retention programs have been shown to be particularly effective in reducing separation among early career physicians, considered a proxy for burnout.

9. **Social Engagement.** Collegial relationships are a major source of satisfaction for physicians. Although physicians relish clinical autonomy, they also appreciate a workplace where they can interact and network with peers, be recognized for good performance, and be included in management decisions.

10. **Culture.** Organizational culture encompasses values and behaviors that contribute to the unique social and psychological environment of a business. When physicians do not identify with the corporate culture, the result is a lack of trust, involvement, communication, and responsiveness to problem solving. The inability to comply with cultural norms is a significant driver of physician turnover, more so than inadequate compensation and other sources of job dissatisfaction, such as regulatory and insurance requirements and electronic health record design and interoperability.

The takeaway is to do your homework and carefully assess the goodness of fit before accepting a job offer. Placing blind faith in a prospective employer may cut short your employment and increase the risk of burnout.

EDUCATION
AND
TRAINING

∞

The Not-So-Private Lives of Young Physicians

Who would have imagined that faculty members would take to viewing residents' Facebook pages in an attempt to "normalize" the residents' behavior? Only the Supreme Court gets to decide issues related to the regulation of content on social media websites.

WHY IS IT SO IMPORTANT to scrutinize the social activities of dedicated young doctors? So many are sacrificing themselves in grueling residency programs. Doesn't that say enough about their character?

Apparently, several physicians affiliated with Boston University didn't think so. After collecting data from 2016 to 2018, they published their findings on the prevalence of unprofessional social media content among young vascular surgeons in the *Journal of Vascular Surgery* (*JVS*). The journal's editorial board, representative of the white, male-dominated medical establishment, saw nothing wrong with the study. However, many readers disagreed, arguing that the findings were inherently biased and blatantly sexist.

In the wake of public backlash, two of the study authors — Thomas Cheng, a medical student, and Jeffrey Siracuse, an associate professor — tweeted identical apologies. In essence, Cheng and Siracuse claimed their intent was empowerment but acknowledged that "the definition of professionalism is rapidly changing in medicine." The authors concluded: "We are sorry that we made the young surgeons feel targeted and that we were judgmental."

In their "research" paper, they harvested surgical trainees' social snapshots from Facebook, Twitter, and Instagram accounts. Approximately 25% of 235 doctors in the sample were identified as having content on social media that was "clearly unprofessional" or "potentially unprofessional" (e.g., profanity; HIPAA violations;

controversial religious, political, or social comments; inappropriate attire [e.g., women in bikinis!]; and depictions of drug paraphernalia or intoxication). The young surgeons were chided for their inappropriate behavior and warned to exercise caution when posting to public websites.

Articles of this sort have been published before, but in the wake of the #MeToo movement and other recent attempts to stamp out racism, sexism, and the disparagement of minority groups, the *JVS* study hit a raw nerve. Reactions to it were swift and overwhelmingly negative. Medical professionals flooded social media with pictures of themselves in bikinis with the hashtag #MedBikini, accompanied by sharp rebukes. The firestorm on Twitter forced the journal editors to retract the article in a statement posted, ironically, on Twitter.

Following the retraction, retweets and comments exploded, demonizing the authors and the journal's editorial team. One physician wrote: "Maybe, instead of apologizing to those offended, you should apologize to the research subjects that you helped exploit. The trainees (in your own field!) that you have an obligation to mentor and support."

If one's interest in the private lives of young physicians is "empowerment," I can think of a half-dozen topics more worthy of medical attention and deserving of research — and none of them involve residents in swimsuits.

Improving the mental health of the next generation of physicians *should be the* real call to action. Surgical residents have an alarmingly high rate of burnout, and medical students begin to lose empathy as early as the third year of medical school, which is precisely when they are thrust into the clinical arena and begin interacting with patients. We cannot afford to let medical students and residents succumb to apathy and indifference as they are caring for patients.

Medical trainees are our frontline healthcare heroes. They demonstrated their heroics during the pandemic and afterward. But sometimes heroes need help, too. For all we know, social media provides a therapeutic outlet for their pain and woe. And it's worth noting that the *JVS* study did not conclude that doctors' social media profiles were harmful to patients.

It's time for academic faculty members to stop pimping new doctors and focus research efforts where they will actually be helpful. The voyeuristic behavior of medical school professors should be harshly condemned.

Breaking Point

*The first two years of medical school are intense. I
put my social life on hold and studied constantly,
yet I never could catch up with assignments.
Add national board exams to the work load,
and you have the recipe for a meltdown.*

Dear Medical Student:

Virtually all physicians have felt as though they reached their breaking point at least once, if not several times, during medical school.
This is especially true in the first two years, when students are tasked
with learning new material at a frenetic pace. Just when you think
they can't pile it higher, they do.

I vividly recall the time I felt I had reached my breaking point.
It was near the end of my second year, with clinical rotations just
around the corner. But before reaching that destination, I had to get
past pharmacology.

Of all the material that needed to be mastered during the first two
years of medical school, I found pharmacology the most daunting.
The amount of information, including the need to translate frequently and fluently between generic and brand name drugs, was
staggering.

About two weeks prior to my final exam, precisely when I
believed I was caught up with all the assigned reading (the basic
science years are essentially a game of catch up, aren't they?), our
class was hit by an onslaught of oncology-based pharmacology.
There were oh so many drugs to memorize, including where they
worked in the life cycle of a cell. I felt as if I was going to blow a
gasket. Mind you, this came around the time we were also supposed
to be studying for Step 1 of the USMLE.

I didn't think I could handle it. I left my study cubicle in the
library, walked down the street to the medical research building,

and popped in to see one of our admired pharmacology professors. Sensing my panic, she invited me into her office, and we chatted for well over an hour. The professor was a good listener and she was sympathetic to the onslaught of oncology reading. Just being able to vent about the travails of medical school put me at ease, albeit temporarily.

My anxiety raged heading into the final exam, so I decided to visit my family doctor. Perhaps seeing a well-rounded doctor might help calm me down, I thought. His assessment was "situational anxiety."

"Take this tranquilizer," he said, handing me a sample package of Triavil. He proclaimed it was a "new" medication.

"Triavil?" I said, while exploring the package insert for its ingredients. "It says it's a combination of amitriptyline and perphenazine." I was familiar with those compounds and, believe me, they were not like a typical diazepam (Valium). In no way, I told myself, is Triavil similar to the benzodiazepine class of medication commonly used to treat anxiety disorders. "It's an antidepressant and antipsychotic combined in one pill," I continued. "This will knock me out!"

The physician insisted it was a tranquilizer to help me "get by." Though I disagreed, I thanked him and left the office. I discarded the medication once I got home.

It occurred to me that, as a second-year medical student, I already knew more about the pharmacology of this drug than my family doctor, whose knowledge appeared to be on par with the drug representative who dropped off the sample medication.

I was comforted by the fact that I possessed a fairly good understanding of pharmacology, at least enough to overrule my family physician and enter the final exam with confidence. In retrospect, I should have given myself more credit for the knowledge I already possessed.

Now, I know what you are probably thinking. Comparing myself to a doctor whose knowledge of therapeutics was gleaned primarily from a drug "detail" is bound to instill feelings of superiority in even the lowliest of medical students. He must not be a very good doctor if he does not keep up with the medical literature to stay abreast of the latest advancements in practice and relies on marketing information instead.

I would not argue this point with you. But consider this: There were other times in my third and fourth years when I thought I didn't measure up. I was inclined to compare myself to my classmates — a better benchmark than my family doctor — but it was useless. Invariably, I discovered, I had areas of strength where they had weaknesses, and vice versa. We all are prone to feeling like imposters (see essay 15). Don't let perceived inadequacies define who you are.

Long before medical school, most of us achieved some degree of superstar status in our education. We were well tested on the educational battlefield and survived a very competitive pyramid system. Although we often doubt ourselves and our abilities, we should realize that past behavior is the best predictor of future behavior, and given our track record of exceptional performance, there is no reason to believe we won't succeed in present and future times.

The most influential physician in my life, my analyst, said it best during medical school orientation: "You all belong here." The sooner we realize that, the sooner we can avoid untold worry and grief, not to mention burnout and depression, which beset many doctors today.

If your mood becomes persistently depressed, however, it's a red flag that you need help. Don't hesitate to utilize resources available at your school or elsewhere — support groups, yoga, meditation, mindfulness exercises, psychotherapy, and the like — to prevent or treat a major depressive episode.

The main message here is to never believe you are not good enough. Fortunately, a simple reality check got me back on track. None of us are imposters, and we must stop thinking that way.

If there is a denouement to this story, it is this: At graduation, I received an award for the highest academic achievement in pharmacology. I sometimes wonder whether I truly surpassed all my classmates in the final exam, or whether the heart-to-heart talk with my pharmacology professor endeared me to her and was the reason I received the honor. After all, she was the course director.

Coping with Rejection Requires Resilience

It sounds cliché to say that we must be resilient to overcome many of life's disappointments, but it's true. Most of us discover the importance of resilience through hard times. The rest of us need to work on our resilience skills.

RESILIENCE HAS MANY DEFINITIONS. It commonly refers to the capacity to recover from or adjust easily to hardship or change. Resilience is the one trait that has helped me recover from setbacks marked by rejection.

Apart from a girl breaking up with me in fifth grade, my first serious rejection in life came in the form of a letter — a rejection letter from every medical school I had applied to. I wasn't expecting to be shut out from my chosen profession. So, I regrouped and was accepted into medical school the second time around. I guess you could say I showed resilience almost 50 years ago, long before the term was cemented into the medical lexicon.

Resilience in my case was measured not by how I fared on my first try, but how I recovered from the setback and grew stronger in the process. I learned that determination and resilience go hand-in-hand. Whereas fortitude may be considered the backbone of resilience, rejection fuels our will and determination to succeed.

More important than my resolve to get into medical school is the way I dealt with setbacks once I entered practice — for example, a patient's relapse or untoward reaction to medication. I tended to personalize patients' misfortunes and blame myself. I came to realize that doubting my own competencies was a form of self-rejection.

How many times have people told us, "Don't be hard on yourself."? We nod in agreement, but self-awareness doesn't necessarily overcome personal insecurities. When the unexpected happens — when a patient takes a turn for the worse — it can feel overwhelming.

We should take a deep breath and focus on one brick at a time, a phrase coined by a physician living with Parkinson's disease. He said, "We have this saying at our house: 'one brick at a time.' Keep at it every day, even if it's just one small thing a day, just one brick a day, and eventually it will turn into a path."

Resilience is sometimes simply a matter of continuing to show up and not give up. If it's correct that 80% of life is showing up, well, I showed up. And there is a corollary that is equally true, illustrated by a captioned cartoon in the June 6, 2013 *Wall Street Journal*: "Actually, I've found 90 percent of success isn't showing up, it's shutting up."

Different types of rejection test our resilience in different ways. After medical school, the most common form of rejection is failure to match into a residency training program. This crushing blow has derailed the careers of many physicians, sometimes permanently. Approximately 10% of fourth-year medical students from U.S.-based MD and DO schools fail to match and must undertake a different approach to applying and interviewing. Successful reapplicants find resilience in their inner strength and courage to overcome adversity. They are able to unleash untapped potential when they need it most. Armed with resilience and a support system, it is possible to overcome virtually any career impasse.

Medical students who match on their first attempt also are labeled "resilient," but for totally different reasons than their unmatched counterparts. Medical school graduates in 2021 were significantly impacted by the coronavirus pandemic, not only in their experiences caring for patients, but also by changes in the residency application process, which included virtual interviews, cancelled away rotations, and rescheduled board exams. Melanie S. Sulistio, MD, associate dean for student affairs at the University of Texas Southwestern Medical School, remarked, "Not surprisingly, because of their unique experiences and perspective, these students are incredibly resilient, graceful under pressure, and have risen far beyond the call to serve others."

Medical student and resident resilience is a trending topic among medical schools as evidenced by the ongoing research and program development. But resilience is also important as our careers progress after residency. I have had to summon resilience to cope with many types of rejection — rejection by employers, government funding sources (for research), and even medical journal editors. One journal, in particular, has rejected my manuscripts a half-dozen times, always for the same reason: "Criteria for determining acceptance include priority, originality, quality, and appeal for our general medical audience. Unfortunately, your manuscript was judged by the editors not to have met the criteria necessary for publication." Undaunted, I found other homes for my manuscripts.

Once, I tried my hand at writing poetry. My submission was met with a quick and resounding rejection: "Knowing the frustration of many writers and poets, we strive to give a reply sooner than later. Unfortunately, given the volume of submissions we receive, even strong work such as yours has to be declined." If my poem is truly "strong work," why not try publishing it elsewhere? Eventually, I succeeded.

Whatever ordeals our professional lives may impose, it cannot match our innate ability to cope with adversity. And speaking for a cohort of physicians who have had the privilege of treating the full spectrum of humanity and marveled at the resilience of our patients and their families, perspective should probably be added to the list of coping skills we need to be resilient for the long haul.

Medical Education Needs a Tune-Up

Medical schools are moving away from traditional didactics toward case-based learning, which more closely resembles how physicians deal with problems in clinical settings. Both traditional and case-based teaching have benefits, but students' learning preferences count, too, and should not be overlooked.

MEDICAL SCHOOLS IN THE 1970S, when I attended, used a very traditional means of instructing: by lecturing on topics within individual courses. We were drilled in anatomy, biochemistry, pathology, pharmacology, and other courses common to the biomedical sciences.

This traditional lecture-based learning was the norm until around the turn of the century, when there was a gradual transition to teaching medical students using a case-based method. Students began learning about diseases according to systems. Clinical vignettes became central to the curriculum. Students learned aspects of basic science that pertained to solving clinical problems and answering questions relevant to the case. The case-based method of teaching and learning evolved from problem-based learning and was touted for its deep learning.

There are other advantages of case-based learning too. It introduces clinical material early in the curriculum, links theory to practice through the application of knowledge to cases, and involves learning in small groups with common goals and objectives. Case-based learning mimics the real-world practice of medicine — especially working in teams — and case-based learning has been shown to be applicable to a wide variety of fields in healthcare as well as non-medical occupations.

Indeed, case-based teaching was the predominant learning method when I attended business school in the mid-1990s, nearly 15 years after graduating medical school. It was more popular (and appealing) than the lecture format because analyzing problems that real companies faced allowed students to generate their own insights and develop critical thinking and communication skills. Most MBA programs today are case-based, using Harvard Business School case packets, and require advanced reading and preparation as well as quality class participation, unlike my experience in medical school, which fostered post-hoc learning and the mere identification of correctly memorized answers from lectures.

The means by which medical students learn — sitting through lectures or studying cases in peer groups — bears a strong resemblance to learning to play the piano. Whether the piano is classified as a percussion or stringed instrument makes little difference in terms of how well it is played. The beauty of the instrument depends on the skill and competence of the piano player, which depends, in part, on how well the individual has been taught.

I was taught to play the piano the same way I was taught in medical school: the traditional way. I was taught through notation (reading and playing notes), the equivalent of taking courses and using them as educational building blocks. Practicing and rehearsing musical compositions was similar to memorizing medical facts and minutia; it was a repetitive process that lacked soul. I was force-fed classical music the same way I was mandated to take physiology, histology, and microbiology. I would have preferred playing the Beatles over Bach and Beethoven.

Studying medicine through case-based learning compares to the way children learn to play the piano (and other instruments) via the Suzuki method: learning organically by ear rather than notation, and nourished by their parents and other "team" members. For Shinichi Suzuki, it was all about creating the right learning environment, and that placed aural learning at the heart of his method.

Listening skills are likewise essential when it comes to patient care. As William Osler, MD, famously said, "Just listen to your patient, he is telling you the diagnosis." I wonder if I would have been a better piano player — or doctor — had I been given lessons through the Suzuki method. I had a "Hard Day's Night" slogging through Bach and Beethoven sonatas. My music teachers never took into account my preference for rock music, which could often be played by ear.

Whether taught by the case-based method or traditional lectures, medical students must master a vast amount of information in the first two years of medical school (essay 29). Students must acquire a certain level of knowledge so that when they enter their clinical rotations they are well-equipped to apply their knowledge in medical settings.

I find it interesting that the results of the U.S. Licensing Medical Examination (USLME®) Step 1 and 2 examinations for students enrolled in a problem-based versus traditional lecture-based curricula are roughly the same; both methods adequately prepare students for subsequent phases of their medical education and training. However, students clearly prefer learning from clinical cases and simulation as opposed to lectures. Osler recognized this over 100 years ago when he stated, "I wanted to be remembered for bringing the students out of the lecture hall and onto the wards."

There are pros and cons to traditional versus case-based learning approaches in medicine, just as there are pros and cons to different musical learning methods. I believe the best way to teach medical students is to pick from various methods of learning to ensure there is an adequate balance between theory and practice, instilling an appreciation for the history of medicine and the changing nature of diagnosis and treatment over time.

The piano has features of both percussion and stringed instruments and is unique in that it is generally considered a combination of the two. Shouldn't the same hold true for the education of future doctors? Shouldn't medical students' learning preferences count, and shouldn't they be taught to integrate the art and science of medicine to be "in tune" with contemporary practice? Roll over Beethoven, tell Tchaikovsky the news.

ESSAY 32

We Shouldn't Let Case Reports Become a Lost Art

There is an art to writing case reports and publishing them in peer-reviewed journals. Writing case reports requires discipline, and it leads to refined skills that can take your career to new heights.

MY FIRST PUBLISHED PAPERS were case reports of interesting psychiatric patients I treated as a resident: a woman with thyroid-induced psychosis miraculously "cured" by a subtotal thyroidectomy (essay 9), the first-ever report of myoglobinuric renal failure due to tardive dyskinesia, identical twins who shared the same delusions (folie à deux), and several patients suspected of having Munchausen syndrome (factitious disorder).

However, I was advised by my chairman to never draw conclusions from a study with an "n of one," because there is considerable doubt about the value of information pertaining to only one patient. "Are the data reliable and replicable?" he asked. "Is the conclusion generalizable to other patients and populations?"

True to form, in 1984, the *American Journal of Psychiatry* decided not to publish case reports apart from brief letters to the editor deemed to have unique educational value. Other journals followed suit.

Around the turn of the century, there was backlash against the suppression of case reports. The demand for their publication increased, leading to cases reported as "clinical conferences," "perspectives," and "hindsight." The development of online publishing cemented the resumption of single-case reporting, with the *British Medical Journal* paving the way.

The time was also ripe for narrative medicine writing "to acknowledge, absorb, interpret, and act on the stories and plights of others," according to Rita Charon, MD (see Afterword). Psychiatry witnessed a resurgence in single-subject research in psychotherapy process and outcomes. The individual case report became a powerful tool to illustrate complex clinical decision-making relevant to the practice of holistic and evidence-based medicine.

However, the rules of evidence-based medicine relegated case reports to the lowest level in the hierarchy of studies. Evidence gathered from randomized clinical trials and meta-analyses was given much more weight than information gleaned from case studies. I stood by the case report as an important source of knowledge for clinicians in their quest to better understand their patients' diagnoses and treatment options.

The learning that occurs by reading a case report is derived not only from the presentation of the case — often a *forme fruste* — but also from the case discussion. The discussion is typically enriched by an extensive search of the medical literature. The bibliography further invites clinicians to read the references to gain a deeper understanding of the clinical issues.

My flirtation with case reports was purely accidental. In my final year of medical school, while doing an elective rotation in psychiatry, I encountered a patient who seemed to have a severe infection. She was stiff, sweating, febrile, and not fully oriented. *Why was she admitted to the psych unit?* I wondered. The referring physician included a brief note saying the patient had recently received quite a bit of antipsychotic medication for an unknown type of psychosis.

The admission note wasn't much to go on, which in itself piqued my interest. Additionally, I was beginning to develop an awareness of harmful side effects of psychiatric medications. So, I visited the medical school librarian (circa 1980, pre-Google), who kindly conducted a computerized literature search using the patient's symptoms as search terms.

The search yielded only one relevant article: a summary of literature, consisting of about 60 cases, of a condition called "neuroleptic malignant syndrome" (NMS). The hallmark symptoms of NMS were nearly identical to those of my patient: rigidity, hyperthermia, autonomic dysfunction, and altered mental status.

Moreover, the author of the article was a psychiatrist practicing at the Veterans Affairs (VA) hospital in my hometown of Philadelphia. What a fortunate coincidence! I called him and explained the nature of the case. He recommended that I withhold all psychotropic medication and treat the patient supportively. I followed his advice, and the patient recovered in about a week.

I wrote a paper describing the diagnosis and treatment of NMS, and it won second place in a residents' writing competition sponsored by the Philadelphia County Medical Society. The case was eventually published in *Psychiatric Annals*, along with another case of NMS I encountered during my residency.

I arranged a meeting with the VA psychiatrist and proposed the idea for a book about NMS and related conditions, such as heatstroke, malignant hyperthermia, serotonin syndrome, and others. The book was well received, and a second edition was published 14 years later as new information and research became available.

Today, the symptoms of NMS are stated as a precaution in virtually all journal advertisements and television commercials marketing medication for depression, bipolar disorder, and schizophrenia. It is gratifying to know that alerting patients to this serious condition was sparked by a single case report culminating in a textbook.

Contrary to medical advice, I sometimes urge medical students and residents to "look for zebras," or at least research and write about patients with mysterious illnesses or conditions that thwart them. Writing case reports should not become a lost art. Including case reports as publications in one's CV will command attention in competitive residency and job markets.

To be publication worthy, case reports should include the patient's informed consent and fulfill one or more of the following criteria:

- Establish a clear purpose and elucidate teaching points or "takeaways."
- Describe a "first" or something new and unique — for example, a disease or observation.
- Report unusual therapeutic drug effects.

- Alert clinicians to serious, potentially fatal, adverse reactions and complications.
- Provide a useful clinical pearl, acronym, or mnemonic.

I wouldn't have been as attuned to patient nuances had I not first dabbled in single case methodology and had the discipline to write about my patients. Publishing a case report, especially early in a physician's career, is a scholarly activity that positions a doctor to become a "triple threat": an educator, clinician, and researcher.

Is It Really a Woke Nightmare for Medical Schools?

Diversity, equity, and inclusion initiatives seem to pose a nightmare for educators who are vocal critics of considering social determinants of health and anything else too "woke" in classrooms or healthcare at large.

AMONG THE MANY DEFINITIONS AND MEANINGS of the terms "woke" and "wokeism," the two that capture the ideology best are contrasting meanings. The definitions are:

"The behavior and attitudes of people who are sensitive to social and political injustice" (Collins English Dictionary), and

"A system of thought and behavior characterized by intolerance, policing the speech of others and proving one's own superiority by denouncing others" (*Psychology Today*).

The first implies a benevolent society that is tolerant of different viewpoints and considers its citizens' race, religion, ethnicity, gender identity, culture, and other personal attributes. The latter implies a militant society bent on censorship due to beliefs and demographics that differ from the individual claiming wokeness.

Why is this distinction important? Because medical schools are revamping their curricula, excising long-taught misconceptions about race and gender and physical health. Specifically, medical education is being supplemented by diversity, equity, and inclusion (DEI) competencies. These competencies are being taught to students and faculty across academic medical institutions in the United States.

At the same time, in line with the U.S. Supreme Court striking down affirmative action college admissions, there is a movement to ban DEI initiatives and defund DEI programs at state universities. Lawmakers want to dismantle DEI on campus in at least three different ways: striking down diversity statements used for hiring or promotions, ending required social curriculum, and eliminating offices in charge of facilitating diversity efforts. Several have said diversity programs breed division.

Those who oppose teaching DEI tenets have been quite vocal and are gaining traction. They are the ones shouting and writing "woke" to suppress educators who in favor of teaching DEI competencies in the belief that there should be no limits on discussing gender and race in classrooms. Proponents of DEI argue that any attempts to dictate language use from above (say, by the government) are oppressive and futile.

To gain a sense of how polarizing DEI education has become, read a few comments to the many op-eds published for and against DEI competencies being taught in medical schools. I collected a sample of comments in response to the *New York Post* editorial "Top med school putting wokeism ahead of giving America good doctors" (September 2, 2022) The comments represent diverse opinions, and I have arbitrarily categorized them as follows:

Beneficence woke

"The idea that humility and empathy are unimportant in rendering the best care to patients is exactly what is wrong with medicine in America. While excellence in science is necessary, ignoring the importance of concern for the welfare of the people we serve is antithetical to the principles of medicine since the time of Maimonides. This includes marginalized and underserved people."

Pluralistically woke

"[A]nti-racism means equitable care for EVERYONE who walks through and reduced barriers to care for everyone who lacks the capability to walk through. That includes EVERY person of EVERY skin color and background and of EVERY ideology and political belief, and therefore INCLUDES YOU."

Selectively woke

"I guess from now on, I have to find out what medical school my doctor went to and when so I can try to eliminate those who majored in Woke instead of Medicine."

Politically woke

"The Left's 'long walk through the institutions of power' has become a full-on sprint... If fascism does come to America, it will arrive under the guise of anti-fascism."

Progressively woke

"What is being woke and wokeism besides making sure every individual in this world is heard and their opinion matters, no matter how small... The sooner we realize this, the faster we could progress as a society, not regress as per tradition."

Anti-woke

"Medicine, science, education, etc., are only about the best minds, and that's the way it should ALWAYS be. NOT diversity quotas."

Reasonably woke

"There is a lot of research that shows that minorities have worse health outcomes and are less likely to seek out healthcare, in part due to a lack of confidence in their medical professionals. So asking med school applicants how they might address these challenges seems completely reasonable. You don't have to be woke to think we all deserve quality care."

Historically woke

"Soon, they will be asking the patients the same questions [as medical school applicants] to see if they will be allowed to be treated. Then people on the street will be asked that and if answered incorrectly, off to the concentration camp."

Reassuringly woke

"Everyone should calm down. First of all, applicants are very bright and know how to answer these essays regardless of their own opinions. Second, you can't become a doctor without passing two very demanding national tests, which are only subject-related. Then there's an additional test in one's own specialty for board certification. So rest assured, your doctors are going to be highly qualified."

Competently woke

"The guy who barely squeaks through the exam is not going to be as good as the guy who aces it. Selecting people based on any criteria other than competence will create many more of the former. Nobody should be defending Woke policies, and I don't trust anyone who does."

Research woke

"[I]f you're going to make the claim that 'selecting for woke-ism over the application and educational standards of students' wouldn't you … want to measure how the actual patient outcomes for their respective residencies or their respective students have held up over time?"

Disgustingly woke

"As a physician for over 40 years, I am disgusted with how my profession now kowtows at the woke altar. A large segment of the best and brightest future docs will be excluded unless they are able to swallow their principles of equality and fair play, so that they can appease these disgusting woke liberals in charge."

Incredulously woke

"I don't find this [editorial] particularly compelling. We haven't had actual effective, smart, competent doctors throughout much of healthcare for a great many years now."

Realistically woke

"These comments are hilarious. Trust me, you all will still be running to the hospitals and being treated by these 'underqualified woke physicians' and they will save your lives, as well as being well-rounded, open-minded human beings that actually care about others and furthering our society."

Being "woke," it seems to me, is OK. But it matters how you incorporate a DEI curriculum into medical education (what science content do you trim?), who teaches the competencies (managing not to offend anyone), and ensuring their teaching methods are unbiased.

Most importantly, how will the instructor's views be expressed — with vitriol or reason — as the various comments mirror? Perhaps the woke and anti-woke movements could come together and agree to understand language rather than legislate it.

The Decline of Whole-Person Treatment in Modern Medicine

The principles of biopsychosocial treatment were articulated nearly 50 years ago, yet modern medicine seems to have left them behind.

A NURSE PRACTITIONER RESPONDED to my op-ed (essay 57) in which I discussed the importance of reciprocity in the doctor-patient relationship. The nurse said:

"I feel so frustrated at times, by the time constraints forced on us by using a business model of practice. In the 30-plus years I've been a nurse, we have moved from patient-centered care (which is the current inaccurate buzzword for the type of care we provide) to income-generated care.

"How many patients can we shove into an hour to bill insurance to maximize our bottom line? I'm looking at retiring early because I feel I can no longer give the quality nursing care I was trained to provide. I'm now told I don't work hard enough or fast enough to move people through. We no longer have the benefit of learning about and with our patients to provide care of the whole person. When I started nursing many years ago, the aspect that was drilled into us nursing students was dealing with the physiological and psychosocial aspect of the patient. For a patient to heal, the entire person needed to be addressed not just one area."

I've seen this sentiment expressed many times by physicians and advanced practice providers who seem to long for a time when the biopsychosocial model was in vogue. This model, first conceptualized by George Engel, MD, in 1977, suggests that to understand a person's medical condition, one must consider not only the biological factors, but also the psychological and social factors. The value of Engel's heuristic approach to treatment became apparent when it was realized that social determinants of health account for approximately half of all health outcomes.

The following list from the World Health Organization provides examples of the social determinants of health, which can influence health outcomes (and equity) in positive and negative ways:

- Income and social protection
- Education
- Unemployment and job insecurity
- Working life conditions
- Food insecurity
- Housing, basic amenities, and the environment
- Early childhood development
- Social inclusion and non-discrimination
- Structural conflict
- Access to affordable health services of decent quality

It seems to me, however, that the concept of whole-person treatment has waned since the turn of the century. We're more accustomed to practicing medicine in line with the biomedical model that dominated practice prior to Engel's seminal paper. I believe we are ignoring the psychological and social substrates of healthcare, and in doing so we fail to truly understand our patients' concerns, including their needs and desires. I wonder whether such neglect can partially explain the low rankings on key health indicators that have continued to fall as U.S. medical expenditures have skyrocketed, far outstripping those of healthier nations.

Granted, grappling with psychosocial issues is far more complex and time-consuming than Engel ever imagined. But some of that struggle is our own making. It's impossible to assess non-biological dimensions of health when medical offices today are run like assembly lines and patient visits are held for 15 minutes. In Engel's era, most physicians were practicing independently and were spared productivity quotients. They were untethered to computer prompts and automated reminders. Fifty years ago, doctors made notations in their patients' charts to ask about important milestones: job promotions, graduations, and anniversaries (marriage, sobriety, etc.). When was the last time your EMR system delivered this type of feedback?

The introduction of EMRs has resulted in as much harm as good: Computers may cause "alert fatigue," with negative clinical consequences. When important social history is entered electronically, it often remains static, quickly becoming outdated. To add insult to injury, about 50% of the medical record is copied and pasted, making it difficult to find and verify information in day-to-day clinical work. Duplicated text in EMRs, so-called "note bloat," also leads to wasted clinician time, medical error, and burnout.

Physicians practicing in the 1970s were free thinkers and private investigators, guided by a deep understanding of their patients' social habits and milieu. Histories often referred to patients by their occupation ("Mrs. Jones is a 53-year-old school teacher....") rather than by gender pronoun. From the perspective of the patient, access to physicians improved during the 1970s. On average, a patient in 1971 had to wait only 5.6 days for a primary care appointment, and the average visit lasted 22 minutes.

In December 2022, I was seen in the emergency department of my local hospital for treatment of what turned out to be symptoms of influenza A and lobar pneumonia. I was told to follow up with my PCP to ensure the pneumonia had resolved. The earliest appointment I could schedule through the patient portal was 16 days, despite indicating "sick visit" as opposed to "routine visit." A call to my PCP's office put me in touch with his medical assistant. The best she could do was add me to a waiting list.

My PCP is a very good doctor, although paraphrasing the late Senator Lloyd Bentsen, "he's no Marcus Welby." And maybe that's the problem. I'm old school (see essay 23). I'm stuck in the 1970s — me, my music, and my medical expectations. I attended medical school in the 1970s. The hit television show *Marcus Welby, MD*, was spawned in the 1970s. Dr. Welby was a family medicine physician with a kind bedside manner who made house calls and was personally involved with all his patients and their extended family members and support systems, or at least he made it his mission to become involved. Welby was so devoted to his patients you would have sworn he had a caseload of one per day.

When the television series ended in 1976, Robert Young, the iconic actor who played Marcus Welby, quipped, "I knew that it was time to quit when I started taking time off to play golf!" His tongue-in-cheek remark portended a prime concern shared by modern-day physicians about their specialties: Which one affords the greatest work-life balance? However, work ethic was never questioned in medical dramas that aired a half-century ago — not only *Marcus Welby, MD*, but also *Ben Casey* and *Medical Center*. While the new breed of medical TV shows, beginning with *St. Elsewhere* in 1982, portrayed gritty, realistic medical scenarios, they were better known for their ensemble casts and overlapping serialized storylines focusing more on the lives of doctors than the plight of patients.

I guess I'm just a hopeless traditionalist and unable to reconcile the demise of the biopsychosocial model and the physicians — fictional or not — who embodied its principles. Sure, I can pay a hefty yearly fee for concierge medicine and maybe enjoy a less rushed, more personalized experience with someone who knows and understands me better than my current PCP.

Yet, with or without time and productivity constraints imposed by health systems on their employee physicians, most doctors appear to be stuck in the purely biomedical model Engel sought to transform. My hope is that medical educators will re-instill in young trainees Engel's thesis that "the physician's basic professional knowledge and skills must span the social, psychological, and biological, for [their] decisions and actions on the patient's behalf involve all three."

Faking Your Way Through Medical School

Some of us remember all too well the student days of faking it on clinical rotations — pretending we were interested and had it all together. No doubt for many it was a façade to deal with anxiety over patient encounters and practice issues. Medical faculty must do a better job to ease student anxiety over uncertainty inherent in clinical practice.

Paul Simon, one of the most successful singer-songwriters in the world, feels insecure. In "Fakin' It," which appears on the fourth Simon & Garfunkel album *Bookends*, he sings: "I know I'm fakin' it. I'm not really makin' it…This feeling of fakin' it, I still haven't shaken it."

Unlike Simon, most students enter medical school with a strong sense of identity and a conviction to become a doctor. Some, however, become lost and disillusioned, uncertain of who they are, and contemplate specialties other than those they had originally planned for. They begin to doubt their abilities and question their destiny, faking their way through medical school to please others or just to get by.

How do I know this? Because I was one of those students. And in my 40-plus years of mentoring medical students and residents, I can assure you a significant percentage of "lost" students have high anxiety and doubts about getting through medical school and residency. In fact, about one in three medical students globally have anxiety — a prevalence rate that is substantially higher than the general population.

According to Pamela Wible, MD, an expert in physician psychology, many doctors lack self-confidence. They pretend to have all the answers, and they have learned to become masters of disguise, lying not only to patients and other doctors, but also to themselves — for example, lying about their mental health by concealing substance use and suicidal ideation. In the "fake it till you make it" culture, Wible writes, "[f]ake smiling happy med students and happy doctors die by suicide at alarming rates."

Suicidal ideation is not uncommon in medical students, where rates of depression are 15–30% higher than the general population. I wondered whether unhappiness was the reason a few of my classmates took a leave of absence. I questioned whether they would return to complete their education. The answer did not come until I was in business school, 15 years removed from medical school. The topic was the focus of a project I undertook for a course in quantitative methods. I contacted one of the associate deans of my medical school and explained the topic I was researching and why it was important to me. He was kind enough to supply data that I could plug into a Markov analysis, a method used to predict outcomes. I calculated that 91% of students will graduate in four years (nowadays it's in the range of 82–84%). Despite poor mental health, the overwhelming majority of students slug through school and graduate on time.

But my analysis did not capture the percentage of students who obsessed over graduating (due to anxiety or depression), or whether they felt compelled to fake their way through school and later in residency programs and practice. There's actually a name for this state of mind: uncertainty tolerance, or "UT" for short. Uncertainty tolerance is a psychological construct referring to the way an individual perceives and processes ambiguous information and situations. Uncertainty is inherent in virtually all aspects of medical practice, and the manner in which students and physicians deal with it affects their emotional well-being.

Low UT among physicians has been linked to negative healthcare outcomes, including less favorable attitudes toward patient-centered care and increased risk of burnout. On the other hand, high UT appears to be protective against oneself and declining attitudes toward underserved and poor patient populations. Medical students who are more intolerant are less likely to practice in primary care or resource-limited settings. However, the clearest association is between medical student and physician UT and their psychological wellbeing, with lower UT associated with higher rates of psychological distress and mental health disorders.

Medical students will suffer less anxiety if they can learn (or be taught) to tolerate ambiguity. Reducing students' anxiety is important because it is tied directly to their sense of worth and purpose, and may influence their career choice. Anxiety is at the root of many situations where individuals feel as though they have to fake their way through them.

This begs the question: what can medical schools do to ease students' anxiety around ambivalence and uncertainty? Can they prioritize and incorporate elements of ambiguity and uncertainty into an already jam-packed curriculum?

Academicians have offered several suggestions including, but not limited to: (1) acknowledging the anxiety related to uncertainty and addressing it by supporting students rather than attempting to "fix" or "solve" specific problems; (2) holding professionalism seminars and courses that include faculty-facilitated small-group discussions about ambiguity and uncertainty; (3) teaching students about the fundamental nature of medical practice, i.e., some degree of anxiety is natural, predictable, and to be expected; and (4) having students engage in reflective writing exercises. Indeed, there has been tremendous growth and interest among medical schools in narrative medicine writing.

Greater control over and understanding of uncertainty in medical practice lessens anxiety in medical students. It gives them greater comfort, suffuses them with purpose, and replaces thoughts of feeling like an imposter with feelings of genuine worth, bolstering their ego and identity. Under these conditions, the need to fake any behavior is reduced. As one medical student put it: "when it comes to mental illness, a prescription to fake it is never going to make it."

Why Not Do Your Residency Where You Went to Medical School?

Most medical students do not do their residencies where they went to medical school. There are pros and cons to staying at your alma mater as opposed to leaving it. I'm glad staying worked to my advantage.

I READ AN INTERESTING ARTICLE written by an internal medicine physician who did his residency at the same institution he attended as a medical student. In his final year of residency, he received negative feedback from an attending who had known him as a student. The attending criticized the resident for showing less enthusiasm about patient care as compared to when he was a medical student.

The resident is now an attending physician himself at an academic medical center. Upon reflection, he acknowledges that he was grateful for the criticism he received as a resident, because the gut punch ultimately made him a better physician. Indeed, this physician has virtually all five-star ratings.

I, too, chose to stay at my medical school to do my residency training in psychiatry. I had done a senior-year elective at the main teaching hospital, essentially functioning as a first-year resident. So, I knew what to expect if I stayed there for my residency. Besides, I felt comfortable "at home," and I had a positive experience that eliminated any concerns about choosing psychiatry as a specialty.

The faculty seemed genuinely interested in me. I had become acquainted with a few of them, beginning my freshman year and continuing into my senior year. One attending had actually interviewed me for admission to medical school years earlier. Naturally, I developed a close bond with him.

But what I hadn't considered was the possibility that, since I was a "known quantity," training where I went to medical school could impose some risks. Specifically, my "honors" performance as a medical student could have raised the faculty's expectations of me, not unlike the aforementioned physician who was perceived to have been a failure for not becoming the doctor his attending thought he would become. Once people know you function at a high "baseline," anything less might raise a red flag and invite unwelcome scrutiny of your performance.

After cruising through most of my first year of residency, I hit a brick wall: I was traumatized by a patient's suicide attempt, as I've discussed in previous essays. I lost confidence in myself. I became depressed. I considered leaving the program. I confided in two attendings who knew me well from my third- and fourth-year clerkships. They persuaded me to stay. I did; however, I was put on probation. I entered psychotherapy with a psychiatrist I had known since my freshman year, the one who told my class at orientation: "you all belong here" (see essay 29). I found that his therapy and droll wit were the perfect combination for my recovery. My probation was lifted in six months.

The faculty relationships I had cultivated as a medical student paid dividends in residency. The attendings appointed me chief resident in what was a déjà vu experience, because I had received an award for the best psychiatry student four years earlier. With the aid of the attendings, I was able to grow, thrive in my specialty, and contribute to the development and education of medical students and junior residents. I was humbled to be asked by the chairman of the department to join the faculty after my residency.

Had I not known at least some of the faculty as a medical student, and had they not known me, I doubt my training would have been so uniquely rewarding. Without the department's support, I might not have finished training. It seemed harsh to have been put on probation, but I know it was not meant as a punishment. Overcoming my trauma through therapy allowed me to fulfill a promise to myself and my attendings to excel as a psychiatrist.

Whenever I counsel medical students about ranking residency programs, I always recommend they consider their own medical schools' programs (assuming they exist). Hopefully, the students have made a few inroads with faculty who are approachable and enjoy helping medical students succeed. I urge students to seek out attendings whom they admire and can tap as mentors during residency training.

Medical students must entertain a host of variables when it comes to deciding where they want to train. Once they've decided on a specialty, they have to weigh a variety of factors, the American Medical Association suggests: geographic location, reputation of the program, work-life balance, the quality of the program director and other residents, and generally how good of a fit the program is. And as we learned in essay 27, fit is important.

Although nearly half of graduating medical students match to their first-choice residency programs, neither the National Resident Matching Program nor the American Association of Medical Colleges routinely tracks the percentage who remain at their medical schools for training. The only information I found online was a forum addressing whether the residency selection process might favor "same place" medical students, and there was no consensus.

To gain further insight into the advantages and disadvantages of staying at the same medical school to undertake residency, I asked a few colleagues for their opinions. They perceived the advantages as basic familiarity with the hospital layout and function, infrastructure (including EMR), and faculty, as well as nurses and essential support staff. Several physicians believed that preexisting knowledge of the surrounding area and city would quickly enable students to establish a work-life balance and good relationships with patients. The workload distribution between medical students, residents, and fellows would already be known, allowing residents to plan their time more usefully.

The major disadvantage was a perception that by not leaving their home institution, medical students would not broaden their clinical experience, and they would have less opportunity for growth and future practice opportunities. A gastroenterologist stated, "If you train at the same system for med school, residency, and fellowship, you only get to see one narrow approach to medical care." An EM physician commented, "I've seen too many docs who went to residency and fellowship at the same program and they have no idea how the rest of the country practices." However, the fact remains that regardless of where physicians train, more than half will practice in their state of residency training.

Transitioning from medical school to residency can be daunting because it means applying theory to practice. It means more responsibility. It means being under a microscope. Knowing what to expect can help ease the fear and allow you to better prepare for the next few years. This is as good a reason as any to consider your medical school as a place to train. In addition, if important groundwork has been laid in medical school, i.e., developing relationships with attending physicians, you are likely to succeed and become an outstanding resident and attending, should you continue to stay on.

The Anatomy of a Mentor/ Mentee Relationship

In this essay I describe critical touch points in my 25-year relationship with an outstanding mentor. A former president of the American Psychiatric Association, he fought to prevent youth violence and mental health stigma.

Paul J. Fink, MD, was a formidable leader, gifted educator, and great mentor. Fink died in 2014, several weeks shy of his 81st birthday. As a psychiatrist, he worked tirelessly to overcome the problems of psychiatric stigma and youth violence, among other causes. I was fortunate to benefit from Fink's mentoring over a period of 25 years.

My initial interaction with him occurred in 1979, when I interviewed for a psychiatric residency position at Jefferson Medical College in Philadelphia. Fink was chair of the psychiatry department. During the interview, he seemed distracted. He was scanning the room and appeared to be inattentive. Yet, just when I thought he was tuning me out, he would ask an incisive question or make an insightful remark. I believe Fink was multitasking — long before the term was invented — and anyone who knew Fink well could verify that his wheels were always spinning, as if he were one step ahead of you.

In 1988, when Fink was president and CEO of the Philadelphia Psychiatric Center (PPC) (now Belmont Behavioral Hospital), I wrote him a letter describing the benefits of creating a short-term treatment unit to handle the increasing numbers of patients with managed care insurance. He called me immediately after reading my letter. We met the next day, discussed salary and shook hands on the deal. In order to make room for me, however, Fink had to dismiss a psychiatrist. He did what he believed was necessary for the greater good of the hospital and its patients.

Informal Mentoring

The three years Fink and I worked together at PPC were amazing. Fink was my mentor as well as my boss. However, our relationship was informal and never part of a formal mentoring program such as those offered by many organizations today. I chose Fink as my mentor without asking him to function as one; the didactic, dynamic, and interactive nature of our relationship evolved naturally and spontaneously over time.

Many people warned me that you don't work with Fink; rather, you work for him. They also advised me to beware his wrath. The truth is, many visionaries and great leaders are temperamental and opinionated, and Fink was no exception. He had a huge ego and easily felt crossed if you disagreed with him. I absorbed the best he had to offer and avoided the rest. Learning to adapt my behavior to strong leaders has served me well in my career, and it began under Fink's rule.

Soon after I started working at PPC, Fink became president of the American Psychiatric Association (APA). He called me into his office. I was nervous. "Why didn't you tell me about this," he barked, pointing to a book I had recently written about the neuroleptic malignant syndrome and related conditions. The book was published by American Psychiatric Press, the publishing arm of APA. Unknown to me, APA supplied Fink with a copy of all newly published books. Fink smiled broadly, congratulated me, and asked me to inscribe it. I wrote, "For Paul: with my respect and best wishes."

Shortly afterward, Fink's photograph and an accompanying story about his goals as APA president were published in *Psychiatric News*. I entered Fink's office and asked if he would return the favor and autograph his picture for me. In broad strokes, Fink wrote across the top of the newspaper, "To Art: this is not only a tribute to me, but to all of us."

Fink was now in a position to display his wisdom and talents to a very wide audience and champion his ideas for the collective good of psychiatric patients and the profession — indeed, for all of medicine. He was a pioneer in prevention and population health before it was fashionable, all the while continuing to see patients in private practice.

The Fallout

It was inevitable that Fink and I would have a couple of run-ins. The first was when he discovered I had resigned my membership in APA. Fink was routinely notified of all APA members who, for whatever reason, let their membership lapse. In my case, it was because I was not comfortable paying dues to an organization that was using those dues, in part, to sue managed care organizations (I was an advocate of managed care at that time). Canceling my membership in APA created a rift in our relationship. Fink said I should reconsider my "protest." I did, and rejoined APA after a hiatus of several years.

But the real turning point occurred in 1991, after I had been at PPC for three years. Fink believed I was not spending enough time seeing patients and teaching medical students and residents. In truth, he was correct. I was hiding in my office writing articles.

Rather than confront me directly, Fink asked the associate medical director of the hospital to have me removed. Fink wanted to relocate me to another hospital affiliated with PPC in a different section of the city. Essentially, it was a transfer, but I viewed it as a demotion and I rejected his "offer." I decided instead to work full-time for a managed care organization.

Fink actually did me a favor by asking me to leave. He recognized that I had lost interest in teaching and patient care, and he questioned my motivation and career goals. Of course, I did not thank him for showing me the door, but in retrospect, it was the right decision for both of us. Since leaving PPC, I have spent most of my career in industry.

Reconciliation

Despite our falling out, I stayed in touch with Fink. My developing interest in healthcare management and managed care led to my next project: editing a book about controversial topics in managed mental health care. I asked Fink to write the first chapter of the book: "Are Psychiatrists Replaceable?" Fink agreed to write the chapter — he rarely said "no" — and a week or so later his assistant mailed me the manuscript, which Fink had dictated but had not proofread.

The chapter was poorly written and there were many typos. I suppose Fink was juggling other obligations at the time. I rewrote the chapter, properly referenced it to the literature, and returned it to him for final approval. Fink, who was a great writer and speaker, admitted he put forth little effort in writing the chapter. He labeled me an "alchemist" because by rewriting the chapter he said I "turned sh*t into gold." It was a classic case of Fink cracking a self-deprecating joke to diffuse an awkward mishap and acknowledge his fallibility.

As to the question of whether nonmedical therapists such as psychologists and social workers could replace psychiatrists, Fink wrote, "The destructive behavior of a handful of physicians tarnishes the image of physicians, and psychiatrists in particular, and leads to efforts to replace them by all types of allied mental health professionals. Only in this type of atmosphere could the question be asked, 'Are psychiatrists replaceable?'"

The Later Years

Many years later, during a conversation with another psychiatrist who, himself, was a former APA president, Fink's name came up in the discussion. The psychiatrist said, "You know Art, the problem with some APA presidents is they don't know when to stop being president." His comment was clearly derogatory and aimed at Fink, but I interpreted it as a compliment of the highest order. Through the APA and other organizations, Fink fought relentlessly for the rights and welfare of psychiatric patients everywhere.

For that reason, I asked Fink to write a chapter for another book I had been working on about career pathways in psychiatry. Fink graciously accepted the task of writing about his career in organized medicine. He wrote about his involvement in APA, the wish to be a department chairman, the pros and cons of "having a big mouth," and other aspects of his career.

Fink was as much aware of his weaknesses as he was his strengths. He stated, "My entry into the APA was a combination of naiveté and brashness. Seeking office, seeking allies and friends, taking positions and speaking out were critical.... If you want a career in organized medicine, you need the following qualities and conditions:

- Serendipity
- A good mentor
- The wish for recognition
- The search for inclusion
- The training for greater power
- Charisma
- A willingness to work hard
- A sense of timing
- A willingness to take risks
- An ability to use opportunities."

As my career progressed, I continued to correspond with Fink and send him reprints of some of my articles. He instilled confidence in my writing abilities and he always responded positively to my articles, showing interest in my career and thanking me for sharing the articles. He was proud that I had distinguished myself in the health insurance and pharmaceutical industries, even though it was a career pathway he would not have chosen.

Conclusion

Fink was an outstanding teacher and mentor. He was an exemplary role model for trainees and early career physicians. He was loved by many people whose lives he touched and enriched, and he lived an inspirational career at a frenetic pace.

Fink wrote, "None of the important steps in my career would have occurred if I had not had an interested and influential mentor early in my career." To his credit, Fink paid it forward by mentoring me and many other physicians. In his final communication to me on June 8, 2012, he wrote, "I think you've done a great job and you continue to be prolific and interested in the Temple [psychiatry] department."

Fink was immensely helpful to me, and I was most grateful for his mentoring, as well as the mentoring I received from other medical leaders in my career (next essay). Based on my experience, here are some of the most important insights I discovered about mentors and mentees that arise out of informal mentoring relationships:

- Mentoring is a strong and valuable tool for developing physicians. It occurs in a relationship that is voluntarily formed by both persons. The benefits are friendship first, learning second, and career third.

- Medical students, residents, and early-career physicians gain the most from the direction provided by their mentors. The mentoring relationship allows mentors and mentees to speak honestly without insistence that mentees accept the advice of their mentors.

- Mentors should support their mentees and not show disapproval or disappointment over decisions made by their mentees, particularly their choice of a career.

- Rather than mentor through the authority vested in their leadership roles, mentors are more likely to demonstrate their mentoring abilities through "expert authority," wherein their unique and extensive knowledge of the practice of medicine serves as the basis for their authority and the platform for mentoring.

- Organizations and patients benefit when physicians assume mentoring responsibilities. It should be reassuring for mentors to know that their role is highly valued by their mentees who, in turn, mentor other physicians, thus establishing a continuous loop of mentoring.

- Mentoring by seasoned, emotionally intelligent physicians in academic medical centers, integrated delivery systems, and other centers of medical excellence will be essential for healthcare to continue moving toward high quality, consistent safety, and streamlined efficiency.

A Mentor's Legacy in Medicine, Leadership, and Embracing Evidence-based Care

An homage to another one of my cherished professors — not only a mentor, but a leader, innovator, visionary, and entrepreneur.

AT TEMPLE UNIVERSITY'S SCHOOL OF MEDICINE, I had the good fortune of studying under highly respected physicians who served not only as chairpersons, but also as presidents, CEOs, and chief medical officers. Anthony (Tony) F. Panzetta, MD, was one of them. Panzetta passed away in 2021 at age 87. As with all great leaders, he had multifaceted talents and provided exceptional guidance.

First and foremost, Panzetta was a dynamic mentor, open to sharing his experiences with medical students, residents and early-career physicians. He was very easy to work with and keen to participate in the professional development of trainees and young faculty members. You felt as though he always "had your back." He had a great sense of humor, as well. He kept a sign on his desk that read, " If you don't have it in writing, I didn't say it!"

Panzetta was an astute clinician and administrator. In 1976, when the Commonwealth of Pennsylvania proposed a $3 million budgetary cut for one of its Philadelphia-based state mental hospitals, Eastern Pennsylvania Psychiatric Institute (EPPI), he stepped up to testify before the House Appropriations Committee and advocate for Temple's management of EPPI, similar to the successful academic-community partnership between the University of Pittsburgh Department of Psychiatry and the Western Pennsylvania Psychiatric Institute. His plan was approved by the Commonwealth.

Panzetta was also an entrepreneur, innovator, and visionary. As early as 1967, he was proposing models other than psychoanalysis for understanding and treating psychiatric patients. He was interested in social determinants of health long before the term was minted, and he was one of the first to question the costs and benefits of psychotherapy and search for empirical studies to shed light on the issue. He articulated problems inherent in psychiatric nosology, including imperfections in the second edition of the Diagnostic and Statistical Manual of Mental Disorders (DSM-II) — and this was *six years prior* to the publication of the groundbreaking DSM-III.

Panzetta was highly influenced by his training and early tenure at the University of Rochester Strong Memorial Hospital, whose psychiatry department has deep community ties and is the birthplace of the "biopsychosocial" model of medical illness discussed in essay 34. He was a pioneer in the community mental health movement. His book, *Community Mental Health: Myth and Reality*, bore the fruit of his thorough meditation on his personal experience in the "movement." He eventually soured on its future, and his final sentiments were eloquently captured in a short but classic article, "Whatever Happened to Community Mental Health?"

As a sea change swept over the field of psychiatry, Panzetta stepped down as chair of Temple's psychiatry department in 1986. The department threw him a farewell party. He remained mum about his next move. We soon discovered he was involved in a start-up company. He founded a managed care organization, which he named TAO. We believed "TAO" was a reference to his interest in transaction analysis – hence, TAO for Transaction Organization. But given Panzetta's interest in Eastern philosophy, we couldn't be certain that TAO might be an unintentional double entendre.

In any event, TAO, Inc., was acquired by Independence Blue Cross (IBC) of Philadelphia. As healthcare costs were spiraling out of control at the time, just as they are today, the promise of TAO — to eliminate unnecessary and unproven psychiatric treatment — was highly appealing to health insurers. Managed care was unwelcomed by physicians everywhere, but Panzetta was more concerned about practicing evidence-based medicine than winning a popularity contest.

I literally followed Panzetta to his new office space in the IBC building and became an associate medical director, initially part-time, and then full-time. By working closely with him, I learned how business practices could impact care delivery, both positively and negatively. He and I often discussed the need for physician leaders to protect the interests of patients in a cost-cutting environment, because we both recognized how easy it was for physicians working in industry to become trapped between medical and management decisions, wrongly erring on the side of management.

As my interest in the business aspects of medical practice deepened, I decided to take the plunge and apply to business school (see essays 71 and 72). My benefits as a TAO employee included tuition assistance. However, rather than accept the meager benefit, I had the audacity to ask Panzetta for a "free ride" for two years at Temple's executive MBA (EMBA) program, which in today's dollars is approximately $100,000. He replied, "Have you ever heard the term 'indentured servant'"? We both had a good laugh. As much as I enjoyed his company, I did not want to be indentured to him or anyone else. I utilized the customary tuition benefit and financed the rest of the EMBA program. In retrospect, given the frequent turnover of industry-employed medical directors, indentureship might not have been a bad idea!

When I was the medical director of a psychiatric hospital in the midst of downsizing, my high salary put me at risk for losing my job. Panzetta told me I never should have let my salary become a "liability." He recommended that in future jobs, I should be content with a mid-range salary, one that is in line with my peers and job level. I managed to save my job, but in case I was to lose it in the future, Panzetta uttered an Italian proverb: "Sempre aria fresca dopo la tempesta" (there is always fresh air after the storm), which I have always remembered at unsettling times.

Panzetta worked the latter part of his career as an executive coach training organizational leaders. He believed that leaders must learn to contend with an environment that is spinning in unpredictable ways. His views on leadership were as follows:

- Organizational leaders need to acquire skills that allow them to be productive with limited resources.
- Leaders require people skills, i.e., emotional intelligence.
- Leaders need to be motivators and create organizational vision.
- Using interpersonal skills and influence, leaders must empower their subordinates.
- Leaders must coordinate activities and facilitate teamwork.
- Leaders must be able to manage conflict.
- Leaders need resilience to chart a personal course over which they have some control.

Above all, Panzetta believed that without emotionally intelligent leaders, organizations will be unable to reach their full potential or adequately meet their business challenges. He also gave the following advice, universally, to all his clients:

- Be clear about who you are and what you want to become.
- Be clear about what your skills are and about the options those skills allow you to consider.
- Be clear about a realistic plan to get you where you want to go, using your real skills.
- Act on that plan and don't become discouraged.
- Keep in mind that accurate self- knowledge is a necessary first step.

It's a philosophy well worth remembering.

The Importance of Soft Skills for Job Success

Personal attributes – from professionalism to manners to self-awareness – shape successful physicians and allow them to sparkle. However, "soft skills" are not taught in medical school.

Don't be fooled into thinking that "hard skills" alone are sufficient for job success. Today's competitive job market means that minimum acceptable skills are being replaced with higher standards. Among the higher standards are what many call "soft skills": the cluster of personality traits, social graces, facility with language, and personal habits that mark each of us to varying degrees. A review of the careers of physicians who have failed to acquire appropriate soft skills reveals they have been tripped up by everything from business meal blunders to lapses in judgment.

The ability to develop and use soft skills distinguishes you among job applicants, helps land outstanding job offers, and leads to job success. Let's review what I consider the five most critical soft skills for physicians:

Leadership

In medical school, many of us learned procedures by the classic "see one, do one, teach one" method. And they called that leadership.

Although there is no universally accepted definition of leadership, or even general consensus on what constitutes the most effective style of leadership, it is widely recognized that great leaders have several traits in common such as confidence, compassion, emotional intelligence, and effective persuasion. In short, great leaders manifest executive presence.

Leadership does not simply happen. It can be taught, learned, and developed. But because leadership, like most soft skills, is not incorporated in formal didactics at medical schools, it is important to learn from mentors by observing their leadership challenges and examining how they have dealt with those challenges at different points in their careers. If your exposure to bona fide leaders in medicine has been limited, consider working with a professional coach to master leadership skills to inspire, empower, and influence outcomes.

Communication

It is essential for physicians to communicate their thoughts effectively to others. That is why so many job postings for doctors ask for candidates with strong written and verbal communication skills. As a group, physicians have a unique style of communication based on their medical training and psychological disposition — for example, as measured by the Myers-Briggs Type Indicator (MBTI), a personality assessment based on Jungian psychology. Physicians may be difficult to understand partly due to their unique medical vocabulary and MBTI makeup, which frequently differs from patients and healthcare administrators.

A large part of communication involves collaboration through teamwork. Thus, team communication skills have become an important part of medical practice. Successful health systems depend on team-based healthcare delivery that will produce consistently high-quality care. A team that is dysfunctional may result in policies and practices that compromise the quality of care.

Professionalism

Mary Frances Lyons, MD, a physician recruiter, states, "In search work, we are constantly exposed to differing levels of professionalism. There are professional MDs and there are less professional MDs. High levels of professionalism are strong contributors to career success, as it is the major determinant of how those around a person perceive and work with the person."

Lyons defines professionalism in many ways; for example, by doing what you say you are going to do, showing up for important functions, keeping sensitive information confidential, speaking well of others, and taking responsibility for your mistakes. Admitting mistakes and accepting blame while offering an apology signifies a high level of professional behavior and earns the gratitude of those around you.

Appearance

Your physical appearance — the image and demeanor you present in your work environment — plays an important role in your career. Body language, style, attitude, and general deportment are an extension of your appearance. Physicians, by virtue of their specialty or work environment, may be insulated from traditional office dress attire, but they are not immune to the basic standards of workplace decency and appearance.

Physicians' appearances on social media websites have become increasingly controversial, as discussed in essay 28. It's one thing to host an instructional podcast and quite another to post inappropriate or offensive content. An Ohio-based plastic surgeon who attracted a sizable following on social media — in part by livestreaming surgical operations — had her license revoked after several patients were seriously injured allegedly because the doctor's attention was diverted from the patient to the camera, meaning she was operating blindly during those moments.

Etiquette

A standout moment in a lengthy job onboarding was a lavish "capstone" dinner hosted by my employer to indoctrinate our cohort in the fine art of dining. The dinner was held in a private room of a five-star Manhattan restaurant. Our host, an expert on etiquette, reviewed the proper way to use utensils, make a toast, and dress for success. We felt polished and in command, ready to conduct important business over lunch and dinner (tip: Arrive at the restaurant early to confer with the sommelier regarding wine selection).

Etiquette codifies behavior by delineating expectations for appropriate social behavior in contemporary society. Physicians are expected to exhibit proper etiquette in all aspects and places of their work, whether at bedside, the cafeteria, or the water cooler. The point of etiquette rules is to make people feel comfortable rather than uncomfortable.

Basic expectations include:

- Address people by their name using courtesy titles, such as Mr., Mrs., or Ms.
- Establish and maintain eye contact.
- Always be polite and courteous.
- Arrive at appointments on time, or at least give advance notice of possible lateness.
- Hold the door for others behind you.

Now, ask yourself whether you need to acquire new skills or improve existing ones.

HEALTH POLICY

∞

The Value of Physician Leaders to Nonphysician Coworkers

*The issues that await physician leaders may have little
to do with their ability to do the work. It's all the things
that happen around the work that count: understanding
what motivates individuals, making life easier for
coworkers, and responding to their unspoken needs.*

I'VE WITNESSED AN EXPLOSION of articles describing the value of physician leaders to their organizations. Evidence suggests that organizations and patients benefit when physicians take on leadership roles. Many top-ranked hospitals in the U.S. are led by physicians. One analysis showed that hospital quality scores are approximately 25% higher in physician-run hospitals than in manager-run hospitals.

Physician leaders have been at the forefront of the provision of efficient, high-quality, value-based treatment for several decades. In their seminal article "The Value of the Physician Executive Role to Organizational Effectiveness and Performance," Dunham and associates found that physicians were quite capable of defining goals, priorities, and direction for healthcare organizations, and their leadership skills were highly valued by non-physician executives.

In fact, in this study, based on a survey of physicians and non-physician leaders in hospitals, group practices, and managed care organizations, non-physician executives often valued the contributions of physician executives more than the physicians did themselves! Why do you suppose the physicians tended to underestimate the value of their contributions?

The authors of the study had no explanation. I think one possibility is that, although nearly all physicians consider themselves to be leaders, they do not necessarily consider themselves to be executives.

Another possibility is that, in certain situations, physician leaders may feel misunderstood or devalued by their business counterparts.

I have observed that physicians in administrative positions occasionally find themselves on the defensive, having to explain their leadership and management abilities to non-medical healthcare leaders, even though one might think their skills and competencies were obvious and essential. This unfortunate situation existed when I was employed in the pharmaceutical industry.

Pharmaceutical physicians who worked in watershed areas such as medical affairs, as opposed to established areas such as research and development and patient safety, sometimes struggled to define their value and contributions to senior business leaders in their companies. I suspect that some senior leaders were confused about the roles of physicians working in medical affairs, and they did not fully appreciate the importance of those physicians because they were unfamiliar with the nature of the physicians' work, or they were skeptical about its relevance to the company's business goals, or they believed lesser-trained individuals could do the work of the physicians.

When I worked in a medical affairs department for a pharmaceutical company, I reviewed drug advertising, sales aids, and various promotional pieces for medical accuracy, completeness, and clinical realism (see essay 42). This may seem like an unconventional job for a physician, but its importance cannot be understated. Advertising that does not conform to FDA regulations may result in corrective enforcement actions, financial penalties, and sanctions by the U.S. Department of Justice, including corporate integrity agreements that impose additional processes and restrictions on companies. Nevertheless, my position, and those of other physician reviewers in the company, was eliminated because leaders who were new to the company believed that a pharmacist could do the job as well as a physician.

I was demoralized and in disbelief that such an important job would be delegated to anyone other than a physician. Surely, physician leaders with strong medical and business backgrounds — in lieu of a pharmacist or in addition to one — could help pharmaceutical companies reduce promotion rules violations and increase compliance with FDA requirements founded on medical and scientific principles. It seemed to me that my company — indeed, all of "pharma" — needed *more* medical muscle and physicians engaged in marketing activities.

Before I departed the company, I sent a farewell email to dozens of coworkers I had developed relationships with over the past several years. Most of them were not physicians; they worked in marketing, sales, and regulatory departments. I was humbled by the many coworkers who responded to my email with fondness and praise — not only for my leadership skills, but also for my value as a teacher, collaborator, and "professional." One person wrote, "Kick ass in whatever comes next! You are a righteous hombre."

My experience, along with studies such as Dunham's, are a welcome reminder to physician leaders that they are, indeed, critical to the future of healthcare. It should be reassuring for physician leaders to know how much their role is valued by other individuals in their organizations when those individuals grasp the importance of the roles and responsibilities carried out by physician leaders.

So, while I definitely agree that physicians can provide tremendous value to organizations, and I've seen firsthand the transformational powers of great physician leaders, I am more struck by the value physician leaders bring to the everyday people who are the most valuable asset of any organization. They are grateful for physician leadership, and they are not inclined to doubt its value.

Healthcare Organizations Are All Talk, No Collaboration

Despite support for the idea that physician executives have many advantages over lay executives, physicians seem to be working in isolation, unable to plant their ideas firmly in leadership circles at healthcare organizations and accrediting agencies dominated by non-physician executives.

THE MAGAZINE *MODERN HEALTHCARE* publishes a yearly list of the 50 most influential clinical executives. The program honors physician and nurse leaders who are deemed by their peers and an expert panel to be the most influential clinicians in terms of demonstrating leadership and impact. The majority work in large healthcare systems and health insurance companies. Here are their top 10 goals taken collectively over the past few years:

1. Prioritize social determinants of health.
2. Utilize genomics to advance personalized medicine.
3. Address mental illness, addiction, and the opioid crisis.
4. Strive for a wider application of telehealth medicine; envision "healthcare with no address".
5. Use artificial intelligence to improve operations and care delivery.
6. Revamp medical education, ensuring that students are immersed in clinical training from the beginning of medical school.
7. Assist providers in adopting population health initiatives under value-based reimbursement methodologies.
8. Apply modeling and predictive analytics to identify and treat high-risk/high-cost patients.

9. Improve the work-life balance of clinicians; address burnout and assist clinicians involved in medical error.
10. Focus on patient care improvement initiatives:
    (a) Improve care for patients with chronic diseases.
    (b) Help vulnerable populations gain access to care.
    (c) Improve transitions of care.
    (d) Improve electronic data exchange.
    (e) Integrate mental health services across other disciplines.
    (f) Address health disparities and work toward optimal health for all.

Few would disagree with the importance of attaining these goals. The problem, however, is that these brilliant leaders, along with their strategic, often hand-picked leadership teams, seem to be going it alone, working in relative isolation within their organizations and with limited resources and outside funding.

National accreditation and certification organizations, meanwhile, have significant clout and push their own agendas, which are generally focused on the most basic quality and safety initiatives rather than innovative ways to transform the U.S. healthcare system. This observation led one review article to conclude, "Whether accrediting organizations are truly ensuring high quality health care across the United States is a question that remains to be answered."

Don't get me wrong. Healthcare accreditation organizations are vital to the patient quality and safety frontier. However, there is a fundamental disconnect between accrediting organizations and visionary healthcare organizations. They seem to be moving in different directions and speeds, and this is one reason comprehensive high-quality healthcare across the United States has yet to be achieved — the U.S. is consistently outranked by other countries in the Bloomberg Healthiest Country Index, and life expectancy has been trending lower due to deaths from drug overdoses and suicides.

Efforts to achieve national certification standards simply maintain the status quo and do not encourage creativity and disruptive innovation considered prerequisite for medical transformation on a global scale. The organizational time and financial cost for undergoing accreditation further depletes limited resources and sty-mies innovation by forestalling operations critical to delivering care in entirely new ways. Yet, healthcare organizations are continually pressured to go through the grueling accreditation process to survive for financial reimbursement, hoping to gain a competitive advantage through superior scores on usual, rather than unique, measures of quality and care delivery.

No matter what happens in the coming years, one thing seems certain: healthcare accrediting organizations will have to transition to enhanced quality by adapting to forward-thinking leaders intent on meeting the challenges of the evolving healthcare landscape. An insider's understanding of what high-quality, population-based healthcare really means should trump the agenda of any overseer who increases the diversion of diminishing resources at the expense of novel patient care initiatives. To kowtow to these agencies is analogous to the proverbial tail wagging the dog. Isn't it time for the dog to wag the tail?

ESSAY 42

It's Time to Stop the Pharmaceutical Marketing Money Machine

*I worked in "big pharma" for over a dozen years.
I respected the boundaries between medical
and marketing teams, and although I helped
companies promote drugs, I stayed on my side of
the turf. I can't say that about all physicians.*

OF ALL THE CONFLICTS in medicine, the ones between doctors
and pharmaceutical companies are the most serious and egregious.
Consider the following headlines penned by the investigative efforts
of ProPublica over the last decade:

1. Across The U.S., Over 700 Doctors Were Paid More Than
   a Million Dollars by Drug and Medical-Device Companies
   Since 2014
2. Now There's Proof: Docs Who Get Company Cash Tend to
   Prescribe More Brand-Name Meds
3. Pharma Money Reaches Guideline Writers, Patient Groups,
   Even Doctors on Twitter
4. Illinois Sues Controversial Drug Maker Over Deceptive
   Marketing Practices
5. Drug and Device Makers Pay Thousands of Docs with
   Disciplinary Records

The exposés reveal that doctors have become millionaires speaking on behalf of drug companies or consulting for them, helping companies promote new drugs and devices. Over the past five years, more than 2,500 U.S. physicians have received at least half a million dollars apiece from drugmakers and medical-device companies.

Even doctors whose licenses have been suspended or sanctioned for misconduct have been paid. The more payments physicians receive from drug companies, the more likely they are to prescribe expensive brand-name drugs rather than cheaper generic versions. Payments of less than $20 may be influential — even a meal can sway a doctor's prescribing decision.

Money paid to physicians by pharmaceutical companies can have far-reaching effects. Many physician researchers double as clinicians and teachers, so their treatment choices and teaching content could reflect a bias toward a company's product or hypothesized mechanism of action. Biased physicians could ignore critical scientific evidence or, conversely, give it undue emphasis. Practice guidelines, which rely heavily on science, could become partisan to industry. The very science base for the practice of medicine could be jeopardized, given that some editors of medical journals have significant undeclared conflicts with industry.

There's already a problem regarding the reliability of medical science. Many research studies cannot be replicated, yet pharmaceutical companies are intent on finding ways to "spin" the data into a meaningful story, exaggerating the capabilities of the product in the process. Weak science undermines good medicine. Furthermore, it impairs the ability of basic research to inform the development of new and better drugs. In essence, pharmaceutical marketing hinders its own R&D.

All this news is not surprising to those who are, or have been, industry insiders. I worked in the pharmaceutical industry from 2001 to 2014. Much of my time in the industry was spent reviewing promotional material for medical accuracy and completeness. I wrote an article about best practices to achieve high-performing promotional review committees — committees comprised of marketing managers and medical, legal, and regulatory personnel. Promotional review committees are charged with vetting all ideas and written copy destined for advertising and promotion, guaranteeing that the information is truthful and not misleading. I challenged marketing teams and stopped them from overzealous promotion. However, my position was eliminated, as discussed in essay 40. I was told that physicians were not deemed essential to pharmaceutical promotion, even though I argued otherwise.

While working in the industry, most of my speaking engagements were at industry conferences — not drug company dinners attended by practicing clinicians — explaining the application of well-established FDA guidelines for pharmaceutical promotion and advertising, and discussing instances where companies promoted products incorrectly and were fined for marketing transgressions. You could say I was an insider policing the efforts of marketing folks prone to taking liberties with the facts. Mark Twain popularized the phrase "lies, damned lies, and statistics," a numbers game describing the persuasive power of applying flawed statistics to bolster weak arguments. Not on my watch!

However, putting the brakes on pharmaceutical marketing is difficult because there is a scenario that perpetuates itself. It goes like this: academic medical centers are home to "key opinion leaders" (influencers) who conduct important research; institutions turn a blind eye to these high-profile doctors as speakers and advisers to industry because they rake in big research dollars; the doctors claim they are not influenced by pharmaceutical companies, even though abundant research has proved them wrong; and big pharma continues to throw beaucoup bucks at doctors and seemingly anyone else who has skin in the game.

Under the Physician Payment Sunshine Act provisions in the Affordable Care Act, companies and medical device makers must report to the federal government all payments and gifts to doctors. Nationwide, public disclosure of industry payments has eroded trust in the medical profession, but it has not curbed pharmaceutical marketing to professionals or consumers. The practice of medicine has become so complicated and corporatized that transparency alone has not had any significant effects, nor have educational awareness programs and policies curtailing physician-pharmaceutical company interactions.

What, then, is the solution to stopping over-the-top marketing practices? I believe doctors hold much of the power. First, they need to own up to their conflicts of interest with the industry, whether real, perceived, potential, or otherwise (see essay 71). I used to inform audiences — tongue-in-cheek — that as a psychiatrist, I'm always conflicted, but at least I know how to manage my conflicts.

Second, doctors should consult with their corporate compliance officers or legal counsel and seek their advice about thorny ethical issues. Institutional compliance officers are unable to mediate conflicts if they remain purposely hidden. Losing at "Gotcha!" ruins reputations.

Third, physicians, including those in the industry, need to dial up their moral compasses. It's imperative that they be up front about who they're taking money from and why. Doctors have the right to make as much money (legally) as they can, but they must be true to themselves and ask whether these payments and business relationships are affecting their teaching methods, selection of drugs or devices, and care they give their patients.

Fourth, when questioned by patients about their relationships with industry, doctors should engage and answer honestly without becoming defensive. Let patients decide whether payments pose a threat to their care.

Fifth, doctors can report questionable marketing practices to the FDA by emailing BadAd@fda.gov or calling 855-RX-BADAD — the so-called "Bad Ad Program."

Finally, doctors should think twice about attending (or speaking at) that next industry-sponsored steak dinner.

If Simone Biles Were a Doctor She Would be Vilified, Not Praised

When gymnast Simone Biles bowed out of the Tokyo
Olympics in 2020 due to mental health concerns,
public reaction was mixed but generally positive.
If doctors were to leave practice to seek treatment
for depression or substance use, would the medical
profession be as understanding and forgiving?

WHEN THE GREATEST-OF-ALL-TIME gymnast Simone Biles withdrew from the Olympics to focus on her mental well-being, most observers applauded her decision, viewing it as an act of courage and bravery, an eye-opener for breaking the stigma around mental health. Many felt it was a positive step because it reignited conversations about elite athletes and other high-stress professionals and their ability to perform under psychological adversity. However, does the enlightened understanding accorded athletes extend to doctors? If Simone Biles were a physician, would she be embraced or shunned by the medical community?

The culture of medicine does not appear to be as forgiving as the world of sports. If one goes straight to the source — first-hand accounts of physicians and trainees who have suffered mental illnesses — the reaction of the medical establishment has at times been downright cruel, beginning with the medical education of students who were never taught to advocate for their well-being.

Paraphrasing a tweet from "Today" host Hoda Kotb, can you imagine a medical school dean or strong-willed department head tweeting: "Doctor, you've already won because you were accepted into medical school. You are a class act. You withdrew from the operation because you didn't trust yourself...stayed and cheered your fellow surgeons...made sure their instruments were sterilized...encouraged...hugged them." Explain to me again how this would be considered an act of bravery?

Here is one explanation from a medical student with a history of chronic depression. She wrote, "The downside to living with depression for almost two decades is that I have learned to succeed in spite of it by putting my health last. But in medical school, we are rewarded for this behavior. We are expected to prioritize school to succeed, spending long hours in classes, anatomy lab, or the hospital — leaving minimal time to study, let alone rest, eat or seek joy."

The medical student went on to say: "I often wonder, how many students like me reach out just to be shut down? Just as [tennis star] Naomi Osaka experienced with her self-disclosure [of depression], medical students who seek help put themselves at risk of penalty and negative career effects. No one should be punished for protecting their health, particularly in health care."

Given this perspective, it is reasonable to ask: Riding the wave of the Naomi Osaka and Simone Biles effect — the phenomenon of athletes choosing their well-being over rules and schedules that may not serve them — will the onerous aspects of the practice of medicine change? Can self-preservation trump outdated traditions that medical students and residents should suffer in order to instill character in them?

A good first start is to dispel such antiquated thinking and make the issue public. I've been encouraged by the many medical practitioners who have opened up about their struggles with mental illness and substance use and have documented their experience in medical journals and social media outlets. The stories of two physicians described in essay 17 bear repeating.

A psychiatric resident had been hospitalized at age 16 after she made a suicide attempt by overdose. The resident remained silent about her history all through medical school and while interviewing for residency positions. Medical school did not provide a nurturing environment. In fact, she witnessed clinicians make disparaging or dubious comments about psychiatric patients and suicidal thinking.

The resident became convinced that she must lead by example and overcome the fear of what a confession might do to her career, as well as the fear of being perceived as somehow incapable of providing quality care. "If physicians step forward to tell their personal experiences with mental illness to an audience of colleagues willing to listen empathetically," the resident commented, "we can make progress on the arduous task of destigmatizing mental health." Indeed, once treated, unwell physicians have the capacity to provide quality treatment.

Next is the account of a physician (a psychiatrist) who overcame crippling psychiatric demons but was plagued by the shame and discomfort of a psychiatric diagnosis. He feared being judged negatively by his patients, lest his psychiatric history became known. "Who wants a doctor with a history of cerebral hiccups," the psychiatrist remarked, apparently yet to overcome the stigma of his own mental health diagnosis. It's difficult to imagine a groundswell of support for physicians even if they have recovered from their illness unless and until they come to terms with it themselves.

Just as Simone Biles has her detractors, there will always be physicians unable to empathize with their mentally ill colleagues, ignoring psychological struggles or writing them off as a normal part of being human. But if taking care of oneself means temporarily leaving the workforce to receive professional treatment, then so be it. Physicians are beginning to feel empowered to protect themselves. Their acts of self-care can be seen as the first step in protecting and preserving mental health. Being mentally tough for practicing medicine is no different than being mentally tough for competing for a gold medal. In either case, it does not mean sacrificing your sanity. It's time medical schools and institutions were on board with this notion.

Whatever Happened to Professional Courtesy?

I've requested professional courtesy for myself and family members who needed urgent treatment. Given the high prevalence of substance use, depression, and burnout among physicians, a good argument can be made for preserving professional courtesy for those in despair.

ACTS 20:35 OF THE KING JAMES BIBLE says, "It is more blessed to give than to receive." If pressed, many physicians generally believe that — or we think we do. But how many physicians actually offer professional courtesy, taking care of doctors and their families without charge or at discounted rates?

A 1993 study published in the *New England Journal of Medicine* indicated that almost all physicians offered free or discounted care as a professional courtesy and supported the practice. I gave free psychiatric consultations and discounted psychotherapy rates to several colleagues over the years. And when I was a resident, I received psychotherapy at a discount. Today, professional courtesy seems to be a dying practice.

In time, as my family grew, I found that professional courtesy was less important in terms of money and more important in terms of my colleagues' availability. "Fever and ear pain? Sure, bring your child in to see me now," our pediatrician once told us at 1 a.m. in order to quell the anxiety of two very worried parents. Doctors always seemed to be able to accommodate other doctors and their family members on a dime.

That's not necessarily the case today, however. I have played the "doctor card" many times to get an expedited appointment for myself or someone in my family, but to no avail. In a recent example, a relative was in treatment for depression, yet not improving, so I reached out to a young psychiatrist who came highly recommended. Like me, the psychiatrist was on the academic faculty of a medical school. I emailed the psychiatrist requesting the favor of an appointment ASAP, and I gave her a brief synopsis of the situation. I did not hear from the psychiatrist for several days, so I wrote again and asked the psychiatrist to reach out directly to the individual whose contact information I had previously supplied.

One week later, the psychiatrist wrote to me on her cellphone: "Hello, Dr. Lazarus. I understand your urgency and concern. However, I do not have the availability to accommodate your relative at this time due to very limited clinic hours due to research and administrative duties." The reply went on to say that I should call the "intake line" for help, and that her colleagues are "fantastic." I was also given the phone number of a facility to contact 90 miles away.

I was dismayed by the psychiatrist's impersonal and untimely response. I felt compelled to inform the chairperson of the psychiatry department. When I did, he wrote that he appreciated my feedback and that I should feel free to connect with him directly in the future, but he exerted no apparent pressure on the psychiatrist. If, had he given her an order to see my relative, would I still want to have the appointment under coercive conditions? No! Either way, it was hopeless.

Subsequently, I had a conversation with a psychiatric colleague — a former department chairperson — about the incident. He lamented the good old days, a time when professional courtesy was a byword and psychiatrists were "complete" because they provided both psychotherapy and pharmacotherapy. Nowadays, psychiatric treatment is usually split between a psychiatrist and a nonmedical therapist — not an ideal arrangement.

My psychiatrist friend muttered "millennials" as an excuse to explain the psychiatrist's inaction. It seems self-preservation has taken root in many physicians these days, and although I understand the need for work-life balance, academicians have a tripartite mission that I've discussed in previous essays: clinical care, teaching, and research.

I also understand there are pros and cons of offering professional courtesy, and doctors must be mindful of certain laws and regulations that could imperil their practice should they treat patients preferentially or give the appearance of impropriety. From my perspective, I was simply asking for quick service — a request from one professional to another. Perhaps even this component of professional courtesy is becoming obsolete.

I remember discussing professional courtesy with a co-resident many years ago. The resident's take on professional courtesy surprised me. She said she never identified herself as a doctor to an examining physician lest the physician deviate from his or her practice standards. Quite a commendable position, I thought, but not always feasible when there is a pressing medical concern for a family member or relative.

The original purpose of professional courtesy was to discourage physicians from treating themselves and their immediate and extended family members. The custom dates back to Hippocrates. In addition, recent studies have shown there is a benefit to volunteering one's time: It helps overcome anxiety and depression. But with the increasing regulation of medical practice, there has been a shift away from professional courtesy to business as usual delivered impartially. Still, it stings when you're on the receiving end. My relative found appropriate help, albeit 90 miles from home.

Why Can't We Say the Word "Suicide?"

Approximately 400 physicians die each year by suicide. Ignoring this tragedy is unconscionable.

ICONIC SINGER NAOMI JUDD DIED at age 76, one day before she was to be inducted into the Country Music Hall of Fame. Her daughters, Wynonna and Ashley Judd, shared a statement confirming her death: "Today [April 30, 2022] we sisters experienced a tragedy. We lost our beautiful mother to the disease of mental illness." An exact cause of death was not disclosed, and no additional information was forthcoming (see essay 60). However, the late Grammy-winning legend had been open about her mental health struggles and descent into debilitating depression and suicidal ideation. It was the focus of her 2016 autobiography *River of Time*.

A year after I had lumbar spine surgery (in 2016), I attempted to schedule a follow-up appointment with my neurosurgeon. I "clicked" on his name online, but I received an error message: "Page not found." Subsequently, I discovered that my doctor had taken his life. I read his obituary on the internet: "Dr. Eugene William Strickland (a pseudonym) passed away suddenly. He was 55 years old. He is survived by his loving family…" However, there was no mention of suicide or the circumstances surrounding Dr. Strickland's death.

Why are we afraid to say the word "suicide?" Usually, it is for the benefit of the family, out of respect for their privacy. But the real reason is that mental disorders remain the most stigmatized of all illnesses, and suicide encapsulates mental aberrations to the extreme. I never considered my specialty (psychiatry) to have a mortality rate until one of my supervisors reminded me that our patients die by suicide and sometimes kill others by homicide, acts which can be prevented more often than not.

One of the first things I learned as a resident — and even prior to that as a medical student during my psychiatry clerkship — was that asking patients about suicidal ideation is an essential component of the mental status examination. I would have flunked my psychiatry boards had I not asked the patient I was assigned to interview the question, "Have you ever had thoughts of harming yourself?" Yet, a myth persists that asking patients if they are suicidal will precipitate the action, despite abundant research that has shown asking about suicidal thoughts or attempts will not "put the idea" in someone's head. On the contrary, acknowledging and talking about suicide may reduce, rather than increase, suicidal behavior.

The difficulty clinicians seem to have in initiating discussions about suicidal ideation has less to do with patient characteristics than it does with clinician anticipatory anxiety about learning that a patient is positive for suicidal ideation. Another one of my supervisors commented, "Art, the only thing worse than a suicidal patient is one who doesn't show for their appointment." It got me thinking that cherry-picking patients by avoiding those who are suicidal is not a bad idea. Then I realized it was not a sustainable strategy, nor is it even desirable if a psychiatrist really wants to learn his or her craft. It behooves clinicians to become comfortable asking "the question" and to become aware of interventions for the prevention of suicide in their practice.

Reading accounts of people who have died suddenly and mysteriously, without explanation, typically invokes suicide as a cause of death. The unwillingness to acknowledge a suicide reminds me of a bygone era when cancer was referred to as the "C" word, and the diagnosis was whispered and discussed in muted tones owing to its perceived incurability. Neither cancer nor suicide is incurable, however. Knowing the risk factors and recognizing the warning signs for suicide (and cancer) are common preventive measures. But suicide cannot be prevented unless we inquire about self-injurious thoughts and behaviors in our patients.

It is more correct nowadays to refer to individuals as having completed suicide rather than having committed suicide. What's the difference? The former notation indicates that suicide is usually a contemplative event as opposed to an impulsive act. Most individuals who complete suicide have thought about it over a period of time, once again providing clinicians and others an opportunity to intervene. Warning signs — verbal or behavioral — precede most suicides. Only when those signs are not recognized or are well-hidden does it seem like the suicide was sudden or a shock.

Contrary to the theme song from "M.A.S.H.," suicide is not painless, but it does bring on many changes — to loved ones left behind. And what about the fate of patients under the care of approximately 400 physicians who die each year by suicide? How do they cope with the loss? Patients are rarely privy to the circumstances surrounding the suicide deaths of their physicians, which often leave them confused and unable to obtain closure, possibly making it difficult to move on with their treatment. Finding another physician I could easily entrust with my spine wasn't easy for me. In fact, after consulting a half-dozen neurosurgeons, I still haven't found one.

Utilization Management Is Medicine's Great Conspiracy Theory

Health insurance utilization management programs appear to be doing more harm than good. The manual, time-consuming processes used in these programs burden physician practices, pharmacies, and hospitals, and divert valuable resources away from patient care. Why do we comply with these programs and allow them to flourish?

THE DEMAND FOR RIGID ADHERENCE to "evidence-based guidelines" is slowly destroying the practice of medicine, and companies that develop these proprietary guidelines are guilty of conspiring with payers to deny individuals necessary medical treatment.

Guideline developers, health plans, and their benefit managers contend that utilization management (UM) programs based on medically proven guidelines will reduce unwarranted clinical practice variation and improve care quality and cost. But real-world evidence paints an entirely different picture. A 2020 survey conducted by the American Medical Association (AMA) found that:

- 88% of physicians considered prior authorization (PA) a high or extremely high burden, devoting almost two business days (13 hours) per week to this activity, along with staff.
- 93% of physicians reported treatment delays due to prior authorization requirements, with 82% reporting treatment abandonment on some occasions, which means patients had to settle for no treatment or treatment other than what their physicians ordered.
- Approximately one-third of physicians reported their patients suffered a serious adverse event due to prior authorization: hospitalization, disability, or a life-threatening event.

- 30% of physicians felt that utilization review criteria are rarely or never evidence-based, despite virtually all health plans asserting otherwise, and only 1% of physicians felt that prior authorization programs led to positive patient outcomes.
- More than half (51%) of physicians reported that prior authorization can impact a patient's work performance, leaving the AMA to conclude: "[I]f PA-related care delays and treatment abandonment lead to negative clinical outcomes, patients may miss work or not be as productive — hurting employers' bottom line in the long run."

The AMA findings contrast sharply with claims made by payers and guideline developers. Improved quality and decreased costs are simply fallacies, a BIG lie perpetrated by guideline purists for years. The truth is healthcare costs and inflation continue to outpace consumer costs and inflation, and the United States health system ranks last overall among 11 high-income countries in terms of access to care, care process, administrative efficiency, equity, and health care outcomes.

The names of the conspirators are quite familiar to practicing physicians. Guideline developers include Milliman and InterQual. The top five payers are United, Anthem, Aetna, Cigna, and Humana. There also are a host of companies contracted by payers — co-conspirators — that conduct specialty reviews in diverse areas ranging from behavioral health to orthopedic and spinal surgery to oncology treatment, not to mention pharmacy benefit managers who have contributed to the crisis in drug pricing and affordability.

It's difficult to turn a blind eye to the disastrous effect of UM on patients and employers. The AMA has proposed a series of reforms to streamline, standardize, and simplify UM procedures, particularly for medically vulnerable elderly patients. But the AMA's suggestions haven't fixed anything yet, and doctors' frustrations are mounting — even the past-president of the AMA has shared his personal angst, writing about the hellish experience an insurance company put one of his patients through.

The Centers for Medicare and Medicaid Services (CMS) has declined to adopt a proprietary decision support tool like Milliman or InterQual, embracing instead a broader definition of medical necessity grounded in accepted standards of medicine. In my opinion, this is the direction we need to take, eschewing utilization management altogether and returning the practice of medicine to doctors, where it belongs.

Do we really need companies like Milliman and InterQual to dictate how medicine should be practiced? Didn't we learn how to practice in medical school and residency training? Don't we stay updated through continuing medical education courses and maintenance of board certification?

We certainly don't need health insurers and their hired guns pretending to know our patients better than us. They don't walk in our shoes. And we definitely don't need to equip lawyers with "evidence" to be used against us in malpractice cases, which is one of the unintended consequences of evidence-based guidelines, as is the retrospective down coding and denial of claims.

Doctors prefer to think independently and exercise their own judgment in caring for patients. We prefer the evidence to inform our diagnoses and treatment. Objective findings constitute only one of many factors that underlie the art of medical practice. Surely, practical reasoning and wisdom based partly on science but mainly on experience and judgment count as much, if not more, than cost-conscious treatment algorithms.

I can't tell you how many times I've heard doctors say they don't want utilization management companies meddling in their affairs (see essay 52). They dislike it when physician advisers — with passion, misdirected though it might be — second-guess their clinical decisions. Of course, there are outlier physicians whose practice does not conform to medical standards, and they need to be educated and redirected. But achieving cost-effective care doesn't require an army of pseudoscientists infringing on our turf pretending to be clinical experts. Doctors are quite capable of thinking for themselves.

Should Consumers Decide the Fate of Medical School Applicants?

A handful of medical schools in the United States allow community members to have a say in the selection of medical school applicants. Bringing in individuals from outside the medical bubble can help refine selection criteria, or at least re-examine the admission process. The debate centers on whether new procedures for acceptance into medical school should sacrifice achievement and merit in the name of diversity.

MINORITIES ARE NOT ONLY UNDERREPRESENTED in the medical profession, they are underrepresented on admission committees that select future doctors. But if it were possible to increase the minority composition of medical school admission committees, would it be possible to increase the diversity of the physician workforce? Better yet, what if it were possible to include members from the community on medical school admission committees? How would that change the physician landscape? After all, we are constantly hearing how patients prefer to see a doctor who looks and talks like them and shares a similar cultural background. Black, Latinx, and Native American residents make up 30% of the population, but just under 9% of practicing physicians.

Even without members from the community, the fact is, recently matriculated and graduated medical school classes have become increasingly demographically and socioeconomically diverse, with greater representation of women and racial and ethnic groups. Insofar as a diverse physician population can better serve the diverse patient population in the United States, it is understandable why admission committees go to such great lengths to recruit students from various backgrounds and walks of life.

The idea of incorporating individuals from the community to serve on medical school admission committees is intriguing. My alma mater, the Lewis Katz School of Medicine at Temple University in Philadelphia, is leading the way. As reported in the *Philadelphia Inquirer* (July 10, 2022) and a Temple news release, five people who live and/or work in the community surrounding the impoverished North Philadelphia medical school campus and its hospital helped interview hundreds of candidates for the medical school class that matriculated in 2023. And one of those members, a 33-year-old youth mentor and PhD student in Temple's Department of Geography and Urban Studies, was a decision maker on the 25-member admission committee, along with medical school faculty and physicians.

Medical school partnerships with community members are not novel; they generally exist to improve the health of the community. People with lived experience in the community may be able to identify social barriers to health and suggest solutions. However, direct partnerships with admission committees are rare. Temple is the only medical school I know of to incorporate long-time residents or neighborhood advocates on its committee. The community interviewers total more than 30 years of experience living or working around Temple, and they often have social service backgrounds.

Medical schools need to ensure a diverse student body to carry out their community missions and strengthen their capacity to treat underserved populations locally. In Temple's case, 86% of hospitalized patients have government health insurance, either Medicare or Medicaid, according to a hospital report. Two-thirds of those who live in the hospital's service area are black or Hispanic, and the median household income is $35,405. It's no surprise that Temple has one of the most diverse medical student bodies in the country — tied at number six, according to U.S. News & World Report rankings in 2022.

The community members Temple asked to be part of the admission process received interview training, and for about seven months participated in virtual interviews with candidates that took about four hours a week. Prospective students were asked why they chose Temple, what community means to them, how they would engage with marginalized groups and communities suffering disparities, and how they would handle sensitive clinical interactions such as end-of-life conversations with family members. Community members were also attuned to whether candidates' answers seemed genuine or rehearsed.

Until the U.S. Supreme Court ended the practice of "race conscious" college admissions, race and ethnicity definitely factored into medical school applications, making it an incredibly hot topic. Some individuals worry about minority underrepresentation while others are concerned about students who seem to be "overrepresented" in medicine. The latter are primarily white and Asian American (e.g., Chinese American, Korean American, Indian American) and may receive greater scrutiny than applicants from other ethnic or racial backgrounds in order to prevent their influx into medicine.

Despite what is now an essentially colorblind admissions process, race may already be known prior to admission. A medical school applicants' race is plainly visible to admissions officers who conduct interviews, whether face-to-face or by video. Even in applicants who are not selected for interviews, many elements pertaining to their identity, including race and ethnicity, can be inferred from their applications, sometimes from their names and often through self-revelatory essays.

The addition of community members to medical schools' admission committees raises some concerns too. What makes these individuals qualified to judge the accomplishments and merits of medical school applicants? How will members from the community be reached, and will the process be fair and equitable? What will be the criteria for their selection? What biases, if any, do community members bring to the discussion? Will they be tougher on their assessments of non-minority students applying for admission? Will their recommendations attempt to compensate for the fact that black doctors are forced out of residency training programs more often than white residents? How will community interviewers deal with the reality that medical students' career priorities may not include practicing primary care medicine in their backyard? And will candidates be truthful about their career aspirations, or will they be intimidated and lie?

The inclusion of community members in medical schools' admission committees is a bold experiment and work in progress. The initial experience at Temple has been overwhelmingly positive. About 90% of prospective students who completed an anonymous survey said the community interviewer added value to their experience and helped them better understand the school. The goal, according to Temple's associate dean of admissions, is to facilitate a match so that the right students choose Temple as much as it helps Temple choose the right students. That's a perfect fit, a win-win combination — as long as everyone agrees on what constitutes the "right" student.

If You Don't Practice, Don't Move, or You'll Probably Lose Your License

Physicians who disconnect from "hands-on" clinical practice for two or more years may not be eligible for a medical license in some states. State medical boards need to recognize that "medical practice" may include, for example, physicians working in the fields of preventive medicine, pharmaceutical medicine, and other health-related endeavors. Medical practice is becoming increasingly complex and diverse and has moved beyond archaic depictions found in legal statutes.

I MENTION IN ESSAY 21 that I lost interest in practicing medicine soon after my residency. I saw portents of clinical practice as it exists today: impersonal, with electronic records and assembly-line labor heralding the movement to institutional employment over private practice.

But it was also my genuine interest in population health and pharmaceutical medicine that propelled me into a nonclinical career. The jobs I chose in this millennium were with health insurance and pharmaceutical companies, where medical licenses were optional, at least in pharma. Nevertheless, I maintained an active license in Pennsylvania, where I worked most of my career.

I relocated to Florida in 2014 and applied for a medical license. I was under the impression my Pennsylvania license would be reciprocal in the Sunshine State. I was wrong. In order to become licensed in Florida, I had to demonstrate active participation in medical practice for at least two of the previous four years. I hadn't seen a patient in more than 10 years. Storm clouds threatened my employment in the sunshine.

I completed the licensing application, including my practice history, and sent it off to Tallahassee (the state capital). I received a letter summoning me to appear before the medical board to discuss my clinical experience. Scores of physicians attended the medical board's credentialing committee meeting. Most of the physicians were accompanied by their attorneys, pleading to have their licenses reinstated following revocation for criminal offenses. I came alone.

"Dr. Lazarus," a board member said, "how long has it been since you last practiced medicine?" I answered that it was over a decade since I had seen a patient face-to-face. The audience gasped (everyone was privy to everyone else's testimony). In my defense, I explained that I had no intention of practicing medicine in Florida, that I intended to work in industry, and that I maintained a license in Pennsylvania as well as a medical school faculty appointment with a well-established record of presentations and publications.

The medical board was not impressed. They said my faculty appointment was an adjunct appointment and that it did not involve medical practice or supervising residents. They did not consider my job in industry tantamount to the practice of medicine, even though I went into detail about how my work incorporated clinical elements related to patient safety and treatment efficacy.

I sensed I was losing the battle. I made one last attempt to persuade the board. I told them it was ironic that physicians like me working in non-clinical positions might be forced to go without a license, yet state medical boards could discipline them for egregious behavior, which meant that licensing boards did, at times, provide non-traditional physicians a license and consider them engaged in practice. "You can't have it both ways," I pleaded.

The Florida medical board was not swayed by my logic. "Dr. Lazarus," the committee member continued, "if you want a Florida medical license, you'll have to retake your specialty boards [in psychiatry] to prove your competence."

"But I passed my boards in 1986 and was granted lifetime certification," I countered. The medical board, however, wanted additional assurance beyond lifetime certification, a faculty appointment, and achievements and accomplishments outlined in my 30-page curriculum vitae. So, I took a weekend crash course in New York to prepare for the boards and passed them again. I received a Florida license, but it was not issued until a year after my initial application.

Surprisingly, retaking and passing the boards triggered maintenance of certification (MOC) requirements. The organization that issued my lifetime certification, The American Board of Psychiatry and Neurology (ABPN), was unwilling to waive the MOC requirement. I tried enlightening them, explaining that retaking the boards was a condition of obtaining a Florida medical license. Still, ABPN was unmoved by my circumstances. They said if I failed to maintain certification, my official record would read "certified, MOC not met." Huh?

I asked ABPN, "What if I had taken my psych boards on my own initiative, just to prove to myself I still have what it takes to be a psychiatrist?" I received the same answer: "Although you will be considered to have lifetime certification, you are still required to complete MOC requirements and retake board examinations every 10 years."

How ridiculous! Pony up more money? For what? A process that is burdensome, irrelevant, not evidence-based, and misaligned with adult learning theory — not to mention that the very act of renewing a medical license requires continuing medical education (CME) courses that attest to and uphold one's medical acumen in the first place. Why can't CME requirements be designed to also satisfy MOC requirements given that physicians are inclined to take CME courses in their field of specialty?

Like Florida, the majority of states require that physicians be engaged in active practice to receive a medical license. For trainees, this is usually not an issue. But for physicians in nonclinical positions who move from one state to another, and for physicians on the move who are active in settings that routinely do not involve direct patient care — for example, preventive medicine physicians and physicians who are primarily in research, academic, or administrative roles — they are at odds with the often-narrow definitions of "clinical practice" and "active medical practice" defined by state legislatures and medical boards (see essays 51 and 69).

Non-clinical physicians tend to become lumped with physicians who have a gap in practice due to illness, sabbaticals, parenthood, disenfranchisement, and other personal reasons. To regain or reactivate their medical licenses, they are at the mercy of state licensing boards' "re-entry" requirements: extensive CME, refresher training, mentorship programs, mini-residencies, passing clinical assessments and board exams, etc. From that perspective, only being ordered to retake my boards was a gift.

The takeaway from this story is to maintain your medical license even if it is not a requirement for your current job or intended line of work. However, if you envision moving to another state and have not seen patients within two years, find out what the requirements are for licensure in that state before you move there or accept a new position. Some states may be willing to relegate you to a second-tier license, e.g., "administrative," "retired," or "faculty," but these categories are generally insufficient for the purpose of providing one-to-one patient care.

"Political Creep": Government Intrusion in Healthcare

The American Medical Association (AMA) is concerned about the expansion of non-physicians' scope of practice and removal of physicians from patient care teams. I'm more concerned about the failure of the AMA to protect physicians against government officials seeking a stake in diagnosis and treatment decisions.

THE AMERICAN MEDICAL ASSOCIATION (AMA) would have you believe that the biggest threat to the medical profession is "scope creep" — the intrusion of advanced practice providers into medical practice.

The way I see it, this is no big deal; the movement will reach equilibrium, and everyone will play nicely in the sandbox.

I believe the biggest threat to the medical profession is "political creep" — the increasing government intrusion in medical matters.

At first, it was abortion, with the Supreme Court overturning *Roe v Wade*, and then there were attempts to suspend the FDA's approval of mifepristone, one of two drugs used in combination to cause an abortion. Now, many states are moving to ban gender-affirming treatments for transgender youth.

Despite scientific rationale and support for gender-affirming treatment by the American Medical Association, the American Academy of Pediatrics, the American Psychological Association, and the Health and Human Services Office of Population Affairs, politicians have managed to throw evidenced-based guidance documents out the window to act on their own agenda. They want to codify their own ill-advised guidance documents into law.

The most alarming developments have occurred in Florida, where only a few elected officials hold the power and control medical decision-making, amounting to fascist-like authority over medically trained individuals while potentially turning like-minded states into medical wastelands of backward science.

Turn back the clock 50 years, and you'll see that "homosexuality" was considered a mental illness (essay 17). However, the American Psychiatric Association reversed that grievous error (originally perpetuated by them). It was never necessary to consult with politicians or seek their approval to declassify homosexuality as a mental disorder.

Thanks to the tireless efforts of a few gay activists in the early 1970s, John Fryer, MD, most notable among them, homosexuality was eliminated from the Diagnostic and Statistical Manual of Mental Disorders (DSM), providing an overnight "cure" for millions of Americans.

Today, it's not that simple (not that it was easy for Fryer and colleagues). The issue for children and adolescents diagnosed with gender dysphoria is not the diagnosis as much as it's the treatment. Florida law bans gender-affirming medical care such as puberty blockers or hormone therapy for transgender youth, and also enacts obstacles for adults to access treatment.

Politicians feel they need to govern therapy, they say, because gender transition may be irreversible, and children and adolescents lack decision-making capacity. However, sensitive medical concerns can and should be handled between doctors, parents (or designated surrogates), and medical experts, like other complex conditions in medicine.

Two studies, one published in *Pediatrics* and the other in *The Lancet Child & Adolescent Health*, both found that most transgender youths stuck with their new gender identity. Florida officials preferred to use the Merck Manual and other dubious sources instead of peer-reviewed scientific studies to make their case. That's OK with me because even the Merck Manual recognizes "there is no conclusive research to guide [the] decision" regarding the medical transition of prepubertal children with gender dysphoria. Why did Florida ban transgender treatment for minors if no reputable sources provided a scientific basis for doing so?

Gender dysphoria is not a contrived disorder or phase of life. The goal of therapy is to align patients' physical appearance with their experienced gender. Doctors who are against assisting minors and their parents can refer them. But before they dismiss them, doctors should realize that gender dysphoria is so severe that it is associated with clinically significant distress and impairment in social, school, or other important areas of functioning. It doesn't require an army of politicians — or any politician, for that matter — to dictate therapy to doctors. Politicians have no place in doctors' offices, and patients and families should not be used as political pawns.

To be sure, there are many areas of medicine other than reproduction and gender identity where the government has overstepped its authority. Martin Merritt, a healthcare attorney in Texas, writes: "Virtually every federal regulatory concern currently plaguing the modern practice of medicine also existed in some form in the 1950s." He cites medical coding, billing, advertising, and off-label prescribing issues.

Federal offenses have grown to include Stark Law, the Anti-Kickback Statute, HIPAA, and the Medicare law, commensurate with Title 42 of the United States Code, which contains civil rights and health and human services laws. Merritt concludes, "Many fear, and rightly so, that as health care insurance exchanges offered at healthcare.gov become fully operational, the federal takeover of the practice of medicine will soon be complete."

Government meddling is nearly universal when it comes to mandated electronic health records (EHRs). EHRs have disrupted and exploited the patient-physician relationship. Excessive evaluation and management documentation requirements take time away from patient care and make it difficult to locate pertinent medical information in a patient's record.

Intrusive government regulations and mandates of various insurance plans have caused patients to shift from plan to plan — and from doctor to doctor — so that the concept of patient-centered care has been diluted and, in many cases, lost. What good does it do to tell Florida parents "to reach out to their child's healthcare provider for more information [about gender dysphoria]" when their provider may no longer accept their insurance? Besides, under Florida law, Medicaid will not reimburse treatment.

Former CMS Administrator Seema Verma became embroiled in controversy, in part because she sought less healthcare regulation and more free-market competition. She was certain that redirecting the U.S. healthcare system away from government regulation would be an improvement, allowing physicians to compete on cost and quality and patients to make their own decisions about their care.

The government's regulation of reproductive health and mental health has upped the ante. As a psychiatrist, I know a lot more about mental health, and what's clear to me is that the American mental health care system was founded on principles of humane treatment and scientific inquiry, not on the backs of political hacks who depend on voters for their livelihood. Where did they receive their medical education?

Physicians and patients were once relatively free to contract for services in any way they saw fit. That adage no longer applies. The medical profession has been gradually caving in to arm-twisting politicians. Politicians now dictate the rules and regulations under which physicians practice. Scientific truths have become inconvenient, circumvented, ignored, or labeled "woke" (see essay 33) or conspiracy theories.

Increasingly, state medical boards have become the targets of political creep. A majority of board members are appointed by states' governors. Consciously or unconsciously, their decision-making is affected by state-wide politics, not unlike the way physicians have been influenced by drug companies. It's all too easy (and convenient) for practicing doctors to be punished when their actions deviate from standards set by medical boards that are beholden to reigning political ideology.

The Florida law has created a chilling effect on the medical community by inserting politics into healthcare. Jeffrey A. Singer, MD, a senior fellow at the Cato Institute, said the government has "killed" the medical profession: "Governments and hospital administrators hold all the power, while doctors — and worse still, patients — hold none."

The AMA's Code of Medical Ethics states that physicians should work to change unjust laws. However, other than opposing the government's intrusion and criminalization of medical procedures, the AMA has been powerless to effect change. Simply put, the medical profession has lost its grip on the autonomous practice of medicine. The American healthcare system is dominated by the government instead of medical leaders and experts.

The sad part is not the elimination of personal liberties by the government; rather, it's that political leaders have coopted physicians and censored those who can lend a voice to patients in need. Unchecked, the government will arrogate the power to resolve thorny medical issues and arbitrarily change medical rules, as I discuss in the following essay.

Stop Passing Off Politics as Evidence-Based Medicine

The preceding essay makes the point that politicians should not dictate medical treatment. The corollary is that physicians should follow the science rather than a rigid framework of political doctrine. Don't let the non-medical ideologues deter you from speaking the truth. Fight back with evidence.

As POLITICAL CAMPAIGNS have increasingly targeted medical practice issues, there have been a spate of articles and op-eds about the apparent corruption of medicine by politics. The American Medical Association believes it is a significant problem, because it is working on a solution to keep politics out of medicine. Nevertheless, it seems as though doctors and other healthcare workers have been steamrolled by the political system into surrendering their autonomy and medical decision-making.

I was reminded of this grim reality when Mehmet Oz, MD, said that a woman's right to an abortion was between herself, her doctor, and her local politicians. It's bad enough that physicians' political views and party affiliations affect their treatment decisions, but do we really need politicians meddling in the doctor-patient relationship?

It's no surprise that medical professionals have been guided by their own political ideology to either combat elected officials or join them, depending on the issue. And therein lies the real problem. We have abandoned science and scientific reasoning to further our personal agendas on "the issues," leading the medical profession into an internecine war and causing further divisiveness among physicians and the practice guidelines and standards promulgated by them.

For example, as I discussed in the previous essay, Florida has effectively banned physicians from aiding in the "transition" of transgender youth, creating considerable animus and essentially taking the matter out of the hands of practicing physicians. The Florida Board of Medicine codified into law its own uniquely derived standards for the treatment of gender dysphoria.

It doesn't matter that Florida's standards deviate widely from those of a half-dozen medical societies and organizations. The point is, other than providing comments to the Florida Board of Medicine, practicing physicians had no real input into the final version of the treatment standards. Instead, those who served on the Florida Board of Medicine called the shots — and we can't ignore the fact that all physicians who are board members were appointed by the governor.

Make no mistake, it is not uncommon to become ideologically blind to science when working for powerful people and even weaker sources of influence. Physicians believed pharmaceutical salespeople did not affect their choice of therapy, but studies proved them wrong.

Do No Harm, a non-profit organization, was a key proponent of Florida's ban on gender-assisted therapy. In a letter to the Florida Board of Medicine, Stanley Goldfarb, MD, founder and chairman of Do No Harm, accused the medical establishment of refusing "to side with science." But whose version of science are we talking about: those in the medical profession who cite favorable outcomes following gender transition therapy, or those who point to its possible harmful and irreversible effects?

The debate reminds me of how two (or more) scientific societies can review the extant medical literature and relevant scientific studies, yet propose vastly different practice guidelines, as was the case with Lyme disease a decade ago. The Attorney General of Connecticut had to intervene to help align the discordant guidelines so that patients could be properly treated. Once again, because of our internal struggles to understand science, its limitations, and applications to medical practice, autonomy and self-determination were stripped from us.

The founder of Do No Harm was troubled by the impact of racial reckoning on medical practice. Specifically, he was concerned about claims that systemic racism is responsible for disparities in health outcomes. The issues identified by Do No Harm on their website and in the news are perhaps the most vexing in medical education and practice today: affirmative action admission policies; mandatory anti-racism training; and divisive and possibly race-based discriminatory practices at universities and medical schools that violate academic freedom.

My hope is that we can discuss these (and other) topics without politicians in the exam room. I want to engage in passionate (not over-heated) discussions about social determinants of health, the injection of identity politics into medical research and education, and the validity of implicit bias and whether it contributes to microaggressions. I want to hear more from workers on both sides of the aisle who voiced reasoned opposition to what they perceived as contradictory and unjust COVID-19 policies and later faced recrimination.

I strive to be tolerant of individuals who hold opposing views rather than participate in walk-outs, threaten violence, or snub colleagues by calling them "woke" and other derogatory terms (essay 33). "It just tells us how terrible our culture is becoming, that we can't have an honest scientific debate about the things we disagree on," remarked Georges Benjamin, MD, executive director of the American Public Health Association (APHA). Benjamin made that statement after public health expert Leana Wen, MD, was forced to cancel her panel discussion at the 2022 APHA annual meeting due to credible threats against her life — and she's not alone.

Doctors, not politicians, need to pave the way for crucial civil discourse and the resolution of controversial issues that impact healthcare and our patients' ability to receive it -- issues ranging from reproductive health to mental health to environmental health. We should reject predetermined political frameworks for interpreting evidence to explain differences in outcomes. It's time we learned to differentiate politics from science and quash political initiatives attempting to pass as evidenced-based medical principles.

ESSAY 51

The Incessant Hounding
of Doctors

*Physicians filling out applications often encounter a
multitude of questions from medical licensing boards,
credentialing bodies, and professional liability insurance
carriers about any past history of mental illness or
substance use disorder. Intrusive personal questions can
deter physicians from getting care. Why can't we all agree
to ask one question: "Do you have a medical condition
that currently impairs your ability to practice medicine?"*

CAN YOU ABSOLUTELY AND UNEQUIVOCALLY answer "no" to all of
the following questions:
- Has your license to practice in any jurisdiction ever been limited, restricted, reduced, suspended, voluntarily surrendered,
  revoked, denied, or not renewed?
- Have you ever been reprimanded by a state licensing agency, or
  are any of these actions pending with respect to your license; are
  you under investigation by any licensing or regulatory agency?
- Has your professional employment or membership in a
  professional organization ever been subject to disciplinary
  proceedings, denied, limited, restricted, reduced, suspended,
  revoked, not renewed, or voluntarily relinquished during or
  under threat of termination for any reason?
- Has your Drug Enforcement Agency registration or other controlled substance authorization ever been limited, restricted,
  reduced, suspended, revoked, denied, or not renewed, or
  have you voluntarily surrendered or limited your registration
  during or under threat of investigation or are any such actions
  pending?

- Have you ever been sanctioned or suspended by Medicare or Medicaid?
- Have you ever been reported to the National Practitioner Data Bank?
- Have you ever been convicted of a felony or misdemeanor, or are you under investigation with respect to such conduct?
- Has a professional liability claim ever been assessed against you, or are there any professional liability cases pending against you?
- Has any liability insurance carrier canceled, refused coverage, or rated up because of unusual risk, or have any procedures been excluded from your coverage?
- Do you currently have, or have you ever been treated for, any medical, chemical dependency, or psychiatric conditions that might adversely affect your ability to practice medicine or surgery or perform the essential function of your position?
- Have your hospital or clinic privileges ever been limited, restricted, reduced, suspended, revoked, denied, or not renewed, or have you voluntarily surrendered or limited your privileges during or under the threat of an investigation, or are any such actions pending?
- Have you voluntarily or involuntarily withdrawn or been suspended from any professional organization or society; or internship, residency, or fellowship training program?
- Has there been any incident(s) in which you have involuntarily or voluntarily withdrawn your application for appointment, clinical privileges, or reappointment before a decision was made by a professional organization or society; or hospital or health care facility's governing board?

If you can truthfully answer "no" to all these questions, then you are probably in the minority, according to physician advocate, advisor, and author Pamela Wible, MD. She says doctors are trained to "lie to avoid punishment and to preserve their job, identity, ego, status, and money."

It seems that various organizations want carte blanche to review our curriculum vitae. They want to probe our background like we're an open book. Mandatory professional disclosures haunt us throughout our careers. They appear on applications of all sorts for medical licenses, membership in professional organizations and societies, and privileges in hospitals and clinics. It's okay and perhaps necessary in some instances for entities to have access to our professional lives — but our entire careers?

Sometimes I wonder whether regulatory authorities are out to get us. Many physicians face enormous challenges when seeking to renew their medical licenses or obtain a new license when they relocate (see essay 48). In fact, in 2021, the Federation of State Medical Boards (FSMB) reported that over 7,000 actions were taken against physicians, and approximately half (3,402) were serious enough to warrant discipline: reprimands, fines, probation, CME requirements, licenses surrendered or revoked, and other conditions that were imposed.

That number may not seem high given over 1 million licensed physicians in the United States. What is concerning, however, is the following statement from the FSMB on their website: "In an age of rapidly developing technology, state medical boards have improved recognition capabilities to know when and how to appropriately discipline physicians..." Uh, oh. Better watch your back, Jack.

And then, there is a follow-up statement about the "tremendous variance in statutory, funding, judicial, administrative and geographic environments from state to state." In other words, it's a free-for-all when it comes to punishing doctors, with each state conducting business and meting out discipline as it sees fit. A recent study, for example, found considerable variation between states in the questions they asked about mental health on initial applications for licensure.

Probing a physician's mental health is by far the most damaging of all questions. Lorna Breen, MD, was a New York City emergency physician who died by suicide during the COVID-19 pandemic. Her family believes her suicide was directly attributable to her fear of reporting to authorities the mental health treatment she had received and that sanctions would be levied against her license and practice. Fear of disclosure about treatment for mental illness and substance use disorders and how that might affect licensure is a pervasive impediment to seeking psychiatric treatment.

The American Society of Anesthesiologists proposes to distill all questions asked by medical licensure bodies, accrediting organizations, and medical specialty boards that are related to mental and physical health on applications to one question: "Do you have a medical condition that currently impairs your ability to practice medicine?" Similarly, the language recommended by the FSMB reads, "Are you currently suffering from any condition for which you are not being appropriately treated that impairs your judgment or that would otherwise adversely affect your ability to practice medicine in a competent, ethical and professional manner?

This approach provides physicians leeway in three ways.

First, it asks about current impairment and eliminates disclosing past history.

Second, the answer does not require an automatic "yes" simply for seeking or accepting mental health treatment. One can answer "no" as long as there is no incapacity to function in a competent, ethical, and professional manner, which is in line with the FSMB recommendation to state medical boards to appropriately differentiate between the illness with which a physician has been diagnosed and the impairments that may result.

Third — and this is a real slippery slope — the doctor could rationalize that mental health treatment is not the equivalent of medical treatment and answer "no" on that basis, but I don't recommend dancing on the head of that pin. The FSMB clearly states, "[T]here is no distinction between impairment that might result from physical and mental illness that would be meaningful in the context of the provision of safe treatment to patients."

However, sometimes creative thinking is needed. Dr. Wible considers herself honest, but she admits to succumbing to 8 of 10 lies she discusses in her op-ed (KevinMD, May 4, 2022) — not only about applications but about work habits, relationships, and self-confidence. Of course, falsification or misrepresentation of any item or response on licensing and credentialing applications is a sufficient basis for denying a license or other privileges.

But physicians don't need punishment; they need licensing officials to back off until their recovery is attained. Most unwell physicians recover, except, perhaps, for some sexual predators. In reality, there is little research on the effectiveness of disciplinary penalties for preventing reoffending, regardless of the nature of the initial infraction.

My eyes start to glaze every time I'm bombarded by questions on licensing and credentialing applications. I don't know about you, but when it comes to answering all those questions, I plead the fifth.

PATIENT CARE

Prior Authorization Is Causing Even More Headaches Than EHR

There are few intrusions into the practice of medicine as annoying as prior authorization — the process that requires approval of requested services, medications, devices, and procedures for patients. Prior authorization harms and frustrates patients and providers alike by delaying, denying, and disrupting medically necessary treatment. This is not how evidence-based medicine was meant to be incorporated into medical practice.

A NOT-SO-NEW EVIL has risen to the top of the most disturbing concerns for physicians. No, it's not EHRs; it's prior authorization of medical services. As most licensed healthcare professionals know, prior authorization rules require clinicians to receive permission from a health insurer before approving certain patient services. In the case of medications, prescribers must get the go-ahead from the health insurer before the pharmacy can dispense the prescribed medication.

I mention in essay 45 that I herniated a lumbar disk in 2016. It was extremely painful, and I couldn't walk. Conservative measures, including physical therapy, failed to improve my symptoms. My neurosurgeon scheduled me for a lumbar discectomy. I received a letter from my insurance company the day prior to surgery stating that my operation had not been approved because the insurance company's physician failed to see the pathology on my MRI.

I called my neurosurgeon in a panic. He spoke to the reviewing physician. It turns out the insurance doctor failed to appreciate that I had an uncommon type of herniation — a far lateral disc herniation. The procedure was subsequently approved by the insurance company.

Did I need this grief the day prior to spinal surgery? Did my doctor need to interrupt the flow of his surgical cases to lecture an untrained insurance reviewer? And what gives insurance company physicians the right to play armchair quarterback and second-guess the treatment of physicians in the trenches who know their patients firsthand?

More recently, my insurance company required prior authorization of an antihypertensive medication I had been taking for nearly 20 years. The medication is generic and is itself a combination of two generic medications. How much money would the insurer save by denying me my medication? Answer: hardly anything. How much money would it cost the insurer if I was forced to forego treatment or forced to take another, less effective pill and, God forbid, ended up having a stroke or heart attack? Answer: a substantial amount in punitive damages awarded in bad faith litigation.

Rather than fight the insurance company, I suggested to my doctor that he prescribe the individual generic components of my antihypertensive pill. Guess what? The insurance company approved it. No prior authorization was required. Is there any value to this exercise? Certainly not for me, and probably not for the insurance company, which failed to recognize how the system can sometimes be manipulated by a workaround.

Let's face it. Medications and medical services are expensive. Health plans think medical costs can be reduced — and profits increased — by preventing certain types of procedures or tests they deem unnecessary, or by substituting less expensive drugs than originally prescribed.

However, as discussed in essay 46, a survey by the American Medical Association (AMA) in December 2020 found that prior authorization requirements can be harmful to patients. Of the 1,000 physicians surveyed by the AMA, 30% reported that prior authorization has led to serious adverse events in patients under their care, from hospitalization to permanent impairment. Other notable findings include delayed access to care, treatment abandonment due to frustration with the process, and an additional two business days of physician and staff time to contend with the hassles.

As the COVID-19 pandemic peaked, prior authorization's detrimental effects continued. Many insurers temporarily relaxed their policies, only to revert to business as usual by the end of 2020, as COVID-19 cases hit record highs. Access to needed drugs, tests, and treatments was interrupted, according to 70% of physicians in the AMA survey, with nine out of 10 physicians reporting that prior authorization requirements had an overall negative effect on patient outcomes.

Approximately one-third of survey respondents believed that prior authorization criteria were rarely or never evidence based, yet virtually all health plans report they use peer-reviewed and evidence-based studies when designing their programs (essay 46). So, is the intent of these programs to cut costs or improve quality of patient care? The answer: probably both. But how can one avoid skepticism given the skyrocketing costs of new technologies and the onslaught of biologics and cell and gene therapies? The first new drug in 18 years approved to treat Alzheimer's disease (a biologic) costs $56,000 a year, and not only is it not a cure, it's efficacy is questionable.

Physicians must also deal with a plethora of low-value prior authorization requirements that, quite frankly, are a waste of time because neither the clinical nor financial yields from treatment are significant.

The AMA has chronicled the injustices of prior authorization — "care delayed is care denied" — and is attempting to scale back programs so that physicians can focus on patients rather than paperwork. As far back as 2018, the AMA and other organizations developed a consensus statement outlining a way forward. Health plans, however, do not appear to be on board.

Psychiatry and Sexism: Gender Bias in Borderline Personality Disorder Diagnosis?

A diagnosis is critical because treatment is based on it. An incorrect diagnosis results in incorrect treatment. Gender bias constitutes a significant source of diagnostic error. Moreover, it trivializes the medical concerns of more than half the population.

THE SUBJECT MATTER OF SINGER/SONGWRITER Aimee Mann's 2021 album "Queens of the Summer Hotel" conveys the plight of women suffering from disaffection due to the sexism of the male-dominated psychiatric profession in the 1960s. The song "Give Me Fifteen" epitomizes the prevailing medical culture — a brash male doctor boasting of his ability to diagnose women in just 15 minutes.

How does he do it? Mostly by not really trying to understand women, because he considers them "simple." The bouncy tune and rhythm of this song contrasts with its bleak subject matter: the frequently harsh medication and electroconvulsive therapy that psychiatric patients (particularly women) endured in the 1960s and 1970s.

Mann told the *Los Angeles Times* that "Give Me Fifteen" mirrors the real world in which women's health concerns are dismissed or misunderstood by the medical establishment. "It's enraging, and every woman has absolutely experienced it — not being taken seriously," Mann said.

This is not her first foray into the world of mental illness. Her previous album, aptly titled "Mental Illness," won a Grammy award in 2018.

"Queens of the Summer Hotel" was conceived for a stage-musical adaptation of Susanna Kaysen's 1993 memoir *Girl, Interrupted*

— and James Mangold's 1999 film by the same name — detailing Kaysen's real-life teenage experiences at McLean Hospital in Massachusetts in 1967. The title takes inspiration from a poem by Anne Sexton, who, like Kaysen, was also treated at the famous psychiatric hospital, along with Sylvia Plath and Robert Lowell, who figure into a song on the album. "I had this idea of calling a mental institution a summer hotel because that just has a lot of weight to it," Mann explained to *SPIN*.

Certainly, 18-year-old Kaysen must have felt anything except on holiday when she was admitted to McLean. She was sent there following a suicide attempt and a cursory psychiatric evaluation invoking a diagnosis of borderline personality disorder (BPD), a stigmatizing disorder notoriously over-diagnosed in women. Although she was told she had to stay for only a few weeks, Kaysen was a patient for nearly two years. Her account questions whether a prolonged hospitalization was medically necessary or was instead a result of an oppressive male-dominated medical establishment.

I admit, I was part of that establishment. *I* could have been that brash psychiatrist. I diagnosed many more women with BPD than I did men, whom I usually diagnosed instead with antisocial personality disorder. I asked my supervisor how to treat women with BPD and he smugly replied, "Art, you refer them" — tongue-in-cheek, but nevertheless proud of his sexist remark.

A feminist perspective of BPD theorizes that women with extreme emotional instability — considered the hallmark of BPD — are labeled as such in response to gendered power relations rather than a pathology that is endogenous to women. The feminist framework links diagnostic inequities to a broader political and medical context: the fact that men significantly outnumbered women in the medical profession for many decades.

Now, with women comprising the majority of first-year medical students, psychiatric narratives that have been imposed upon women can be changed, and the ways in which power and oppression have shaped their views of themselves can be resculpted. Furthermore, new storylines can be created (and put to music) that are meaningful for female patients, regardless of labels, diagnostic categories, or the presumed power and expertise of the physician.

Unfortunately, gender myths are ingrained as biases that negatively impact the care, treatment, and diagnosis of women and ethnic minorities. According to the book *Unwell Women: Misdiagnosis and Myth in a Man-Made World* by feminist theorist Elinor Cleghorn, PhD, "[T]he discrimination women encounter as medical patients is magnified when they are Black, Asian, Indigenous, Latinx, or ethnically diverse; when their access to health services is restricted; and when they don't identify with the gender norms medicine ascribes to biological womanhood."

Yet, the question of why women, rather than men, are more frequently diagnosed with BPD remains largely unanswered despite current evidence for the origin of personality disorders in genetics and neurobiology, and despite suggestions that biased sampling is the most likely explanation for gender bias in the diagnosis of BPD. However, the essential issue is whether the larger prevalence in women is due to a biased sample or a biased diagnosis.

The bulk of the evidence suggests the latter. In fact, medical myths about gender roles have existed for centuries, with its foundation cemented in ancient Greece, and women are still victims of gender and diagnostic bias today. Bias in medical knowledge, research, and practice has resulted in inadequate treatment of women's pain and a host of other conditions including heart disease, bleeding, and autoimmune disorders — and especially mental health disorders. Physicians must make a concerted effort to be aware of their biases and rectify them in order to best serve their patients.

Although the medical profession is working to revamp its practices and eliminate explicit forms of discrimination and more subtler microaggressions, there is a long legacy to quash when it comes to women's bodies and minds. Women like Kaysen in search of an honest and accurate diagnosis continue to struggle against thinly disguised misogyny in medical orthodoxy.

Medical Translation Sacrifices Accuracy for Understanding

Comprehension is a critical aspect of healthcare.
Doctors' use of plain language facilitates patients'
understanding of their diagnoses and treatment.
But the use of plain language comes with a price:
It incorporates imprecise medical terminology
that may alter the meaning of the message.

THE YEAR WAS 1980. I was a first-year resident working on a psychiatric inpatient unit in the City of Brotherly Love. A family had just dropped off a psychotic patient who only spoke Greek. How did we know she was psychotic? The family reported the patient had been acting bizarrely and was responding to hallucinations. However, they left before I could obtain a complete history. We did not have Greek translators on staff, so I did the next best thing: I ran outside to the corner hot dog vendor and enlisted his services (countless pushcart vendors in Philadelphia are Greek). He confirmed the patient had "strange ideas" and was "crazy" even by his standards. Mind you, this was before HIPAA was enacted, and we were fast and loose with privacy issues.

In my era, it was common to depend on family members or family friends for translation. However, very few relatives had the knowledge to translate medical terminology. Who knows what may have been missed in the examination or delivery of instructions? Unless a close family member or invited friend was a medical professional, a medical translator was necessary.

Fast forward to today. Federal law requires that any organization receiving federal financial assistance, including Medicare, Medicaid, and federal reimbursements, must provide equal care to every patient. This includes serving customers who don't speak English, have low proficiency, or are hearing impaired. Without translation, patients would not be able to understand the most basic elements of treatment, including their diagnoses, medication effects, referrals, and follow-up appointments. Conveying medical information to non-English speaking patients without proper translation has been associated with medical errors and poor outcomes. Given that more than 25 million people in the U.S. have limited comfort with English as their primary language, the language and culture of minorities in healthcare settings need to be prioritized and addressed in order to reduce disparities.

However, translators vary in their ability to translate — not just the words, but the real meaning of the medical communication. Even with the best translators, doctors are seldom fully satisfied with the quality of the communication when seeing patients who do not speak English. And vice versa, patients are frequently unhappy when they are left to digest a very large volume of information received second-hand in a short time span, putting them at risk of being ill-informed of care processes.

My experience on the inpatient psych unit presaged problems I encountered in the pharmaceutical industry. I oversaw the translation of a drug's FDA-approved "label" from English to Spanish. It was a labor-intensive task, involving an outside translator and an internal team comprising myself, a lawyer, a regulatory specialist, a registered pharmacist, and a marketing team representative. With everyone's input, the label was translated from English to Spanish. Then, a second translator not involved in the original work translated the label from Spanish to English — the so-called "back translation." The original label in English was compared word-for-word with the English version generated through the back translation. The concordance was around 85%, far from perfect, but not unexpected because of the natural differences in language.

The medical translators faced several challenges. Some of these included dealing with unique medical terminology, equivalence of medical words and phrases, and certain characteristics of the English language causing variations in semantics and syntax, as well as other nuances and idiosyncrasies. Because the drug label is ostensibly written for prescribers rather than patients, its translation is considered an expert-to-expert communication in which accuracy is generally easier to achieve compared with a medical translation between an expert and lay reader.

The latter communication, such as between a doctor and patient or drug or medical device manufacturer and consumer, necessarily entails the use of less complex and precise language. Scientific and medical communication must be "dumbed down" for consumers for easy readability and comprehension. As a result, fact sheets, informed consent forms for clinical trials, and various types of consumer advertising can become biased or misleading because precision and accuracy are sacrificed for understanding.

Toward the end of my pharmaceutical career, I developed a special expertise reviewing advertising and promotion for the public. My job was to ensure that the drug information was truthful, balanced, and accurately communicated. But how do you communicate technical terms, complex clinical data, genetic concepts, and cryptic yet potentially lethal side effects to consumers without losing some accuracy? Can the information be broken down so that an eighth-grade student could comprehend it, which is typically recommended for materials intended for the general public? It can't!

The main purpose of advertising drugs to consumers is to sell a product; it is not to empower patients or educate the public. Not only does the language of drug ads make that clear, so does the tone: branded drug ads are increasingly using popular rock songs to accompany their treatment messages. The feel-good vibe is a powerful way to aid drug name recall and reach aging baby boomers and other target audiences. The fact that television commercials are able to stuff so much music and verbiage (including subtitles) into a 60-second spot makes comprehension of the advertisement very difficult. The music alone interferes with comprehension and detracts from the medications' side effects and risks.

Studies have shown there are clear advantages to direct-to-consumer drug advertising. But as with clinical care, much of the advertising has been lost in translation.

Do Microaggressions Persist After Practice?

*Doctors' biases against certain groups do
indeed persist after office hours.*

MICROAGGRESSIONS WERE DISCUSSED in prior sections of the book. They are common, subtle, offending behaviors and attitudes that stem from implicit (unconscious) bias. Individuals targeted by microaggressions are different than us — different in their look, skin tone, gender, sexual preference, socioeconomic status, educational level, and age.

Implicit bias refers to unconscious stereotypes, assumptions, and beliefs held about an individual's group identity. They affect our understanding, actions, and decisions and increase health disparities. Once learned, stereotypes and prejudices resist change and are difficult to extinguish, remaining as "mental residue."

People can be consciously committed to diversity and inclusion and deliberately work to behave without prejudice yet still possess hidden negative prejudices or stereotypes. This suggests that diagnoses and treatment may be biased even in the absence of a physician's intent or awareness.

The consequences of implicit bias in healthcare can be devastating for patients, causing them to become depressed and feel threatened. Patients report dissatisfaction with treatment and distrust of providers, limiting their access to care and medication.

Medical students, residents, and faculty members are also at risk of being judged unconsciously and treated poorly. Black doctors are forced out of residency training programs more often than white residents. Women faculty report higher frequencies of microaggressions than men in academic medical centers.

Learning how to identify and overcome implicit bias is essential to improving healthcare delivery to diverse populations. Changing people's belief systems through self-awareness and training on potential biases is critical yet difficult. The key is to learn how to replace biases and assumptions with accurate representations of patients free of racial and ethnic context. One way to do this is to increase opportunities for positive contact with geographically and socioeconomically disadvantaged patients.

Although clinicians may not be able to eliminate implicit bias, it is commonly believed that those who are highly motivated to control prejudice and increase bias awareness can successfully prevent microaggressions from affecting the quality of care they provide.

It's surprising that no research has been conducted on physicians after they retire when they are no longer forced to maintain a façade or suppress their true feelings. Do lingering prejudices affect their everyday exchanges with the public now that they are permanently off-duty?

I do think it is important to address this question, given the large portion of the physician workforce nearing the traditional retirement age. More than two of every five active physicians in the U.S. will be 65 or older within the next decade. Nearly a quarter of physicians are considering early retirement because of work overload. If they are anything like me — newly retired or semi-retired — they will have time on their hands and seek new social outlets.

My wife and I downsized our living arrangements and moved to a large, diverse community. To become acquainted with our neighbors, I typically asked, "Where are you from?" — only to learn it was a microaggression because asking someone of color or any minority, "Where are you from or where were you born?" could suggest they are not true Americans.

We ordered many meals online as we settled into our new house. Many of the delivery drivers were ethnic and racial minorities with limited English proficiency (essay 10). Still, I understood them and wished to compliment them. Do I dare say, "You speak English very well?" That, too, is considered a microaggression.

We befriended our next-door neighbors, a young couple born and raised in Manhattan. I was tempted to say, "You don't talk like New Yorkers," but alas, this would have been construed as a microaggression.

While on my morning walk, I struck up a conversation with an African American woman roughly my age. I told her I was a retired physician. She told me about her health problems and her noble family physician who saved her life, "He's a man of God," she said. I nodded silently. Presumably, she was unaware that utterances proclaiming one's moral high ground are also a form of microaggression.

I soon established relationships with new doctors to manage my health concerns. One of them, a dermatologist, was born and raised in Honolulu and went to medical school there, according to her biography. So, instead of saying, "You don't look Hawaiian," I simply said, "My son lives in Honolulu," which opened an interesting conversation about her background, albeit one that she initiated.

There are "microaggression projects" throughout college campuses, speech codes and guidelines dictating what is permissible to say and what is not. Critics claim the pendulum has swung too far, restricting the First Amendment right to free speech and the expression of ideas and academic freedom. As the debate rages on, I wonder whether guidelines for microaggressions will become codified at medical institutions, particularly academic medical centers?

The University of North Carolina (UNC) School of Medicine, for example, has integrated social medicine into the entirety of its hospital system. UNC's "Task Force to Integrate Social Justice Into the Curriculum" document was released in October 2020 partly to have effective mechanisms in place to address negative behaviors experienced by students and train faculty on implicit bias. Understanding and responding to microaggressions is integral to the school's mission.

I'm obviously interested in microaggressions because I'm a psychiatrist trained to understand the unconscious. Freud spoke indirectly about microaggressions when he said, "A man should not strive to eliminate his complexes, but to get into accord with them …" At the same time, he believed unexpressed emotions do not die — they simply "come forth later in uglier ways."

In addition, I've been both a perpetrator of microaggressions and a victim. The former occurred without malicious intent but nevertheless insulted someone (essay 10). The latter occurred on the receiving end of a waitress raised in the south. "Where y'all from?" she asked, taking our lunch orders at a restaurant in Kentucky. "Where'd ya git those accents?" I felt like an alien from the north.

The most insightful thing I can tell you is that microaggressions are different when you experience them than when you talk or think about them.

Microaggressions can and do hurt. We know this from clinical practice, and most physicians have been taught how to frame their comments with patients (and colleagues) to "do no harm." Now that physicians are leaving the clinical ranks, their training and education must follow them into civilian life.

Teachings from medical conferences, seminars, forums, and discussions that have identified unacceptable behavior and instructed us on how to be culturally sensitive and inclusive should be applied to our interactions with our neighbors and those we meet in the supermarket and on the golf links.

As long as implicit bias persists, microaggressions will persist, but overcoming them will give new meaning to "preventive medicine."

Tele-Mental Health
Is All the Rage

*Beware telehealth companies that do not permit
patients to have direct access to clinicians in
emergencies. Companies whose services are geared
toward the diagnosis and treatment of only one
disorder (e.g., ADHD) also raise a red flag.*

TELEHEALTH COMPANIES' PRESCRIBING of controlled substances has come under scrutiny for alleged deceptive practices. Online health companies have been cited for alleged improper prescribing of opioid and stimulant medication for patients purported to be suffering from a variety of conditions, but especially attention deficit-hyperactivity disorder (ADHD). Two mental health companies in particular — Cerebral and Done — have been singled out by the Department of Justice, and are reported to be targets of investigations by the Federal Trade Commission and the Drug Enforcement Agency, respectively.

Federal law mandates that a prescription for a controlled substance issued through the internet (including telemedicine) must generally be predicated on an in-person medical evaluation. Regulations governing the online dispensing of controlled substances have been relaxed during the pandemic. However, the regulations may once again be enforced in light of the decreasing numbers of patients affected by the coronavirus and the ending of the public health emergency.

Many of the new tele-mental health companies are small yet big-business minded and backed by mega investors. Globally there are nearly 900 mental health telemedicine companies. Many providers who work online for these companies often work independently from home with no professional liability insurance provided by the company. They are leaving a broken legacy system coupled with the promise of better pay and the excitement of a startup.

A telehealth "appointment" does not require a physical exam, vital signs, or neurological observation. Certain current and former employees claim they feel pressured to be fast and promptly submit an electronic prescription. Tele-mental health companies have been compared to fast-food establishments, and some have raised concerns about their potential to successfully treat patients at high risk of suicide or those suffering from other serious mental health conditions.

Case in point: Cerebral failed to identify that a patient who completed suicide while in treatment was, in fact, a minor. By Missouri law, Cerebral should have notified the teenager's parents about treatment, but their consent was never obtained. The parents did not find out their son was in treatment — let alone suicidal — until the day he died.

Meanwhile, the websites of certain tele-mental health companies paint a picture of serenity and tranquility, with faces of happy, smiling people. Several companies advertise free assessments, affordable "membership" plans, and ease of scheduling appointments. They provide testimonials from highly satisfied clients claiming rapid improvement. From what I saw, however, statistical methods used to determine patient outcomes were never given. I wondered whether medical and educational information for consumers was reviewed by physicians, as is customary on well-established medical websites for the public.

Some companies have enlisted renowned psychiatrists and sports figures as spokespeople, advisers, and consultants. Among them, gymnast Simone Biles is Chief Impact Officer at Cerebral. Swimmer Michael Phelps teamed up with Talkspace.

When I combed through the web pages of several of these startup companies, I could not readily discern their key leaders or, in the case of Cerebral and Done, any mention of government probes apart from a comment by Cerebral's CEO that Cerebral has been the "target of news stories that provide a distorted view of our outstanding care."

In the spirit of full disclosure, I was interviewed by Cerebral and Done for part-time positions. At Cerebral, I was hired to supervise advanced practice providers (APPs), but I resigned in less than a month, before any supervision occurred. As advertised in Cerebral's job postings, psychiatrists supervise APPs by auditing their charts, along with other measures such as collaborating with the psychiatric mental health nurse practitioner team. I believe clinical consultations directly with APPs — in person, by phone, or via secure video — should be the predominant method of supervision (see essay 23).

I spoke with the executive leader of Done on a couple of occasions. She characterizes herself as a "builder." Because she has no medical background, she was considering hiring me as the medical director. However, I was told by an outside recruiting agency that Done was also pursuing other candidates. I asked to be withdrawn from consideration, not because I was afraid of competition, but because I believed the company lacked adequate infrastructure and was exclusively focused on treating patients with ADHD.

I have no axe to grind with either company. In fact, one study that showed use of telehealth services was associated with fewer opioid overdoses during the pandemic. However, companies must follow the proper procedures for prescribing controlled substances to patients or else stop prescribing them. (Cerebral disclosed in May 2022 that they would stop prescribing most controlled substances.)

Online mental health companies need to make a greater commitment to operating ethically and professionally. Their websites need to be more transparent about clinical and business practices. Important clinical information should not be qualified by asterisks or buried in the fine print of legal disclaimers.

Consumers should be aware that online mental health care is not designed for those with serious and persistent mental illnesses or those who experience frequent crises. It's telling that Cerebral provides non-company resources for individuals in emotional distress — for example, the phone number for the National Suicide Prevention Lifeline — and requires clients to hold them harmless for delays in evaluation due to "technical failures."

Treatment of ADHD with non-stimulant medication should be emphasized as an option for some individuals, and ADHD should not be the sole focus of treatment of online mental health care. Providers should be well-versed in the diagnosis and treatment of all major mental health disorders.

Celebrities should think twice about lending their names to mental health startups simply to increase the company's market visibility. All clinical information geared toward consumers should pass scientific muster: The information must be accurate, complete, and not misleading. Companies should make it known that claims of efficacy and positive outcomes reflect only clients who volunteer their experience and are, therefore, not valid statistical samples.

While there are clear indications to treat psychiatric and other disorders with controlled substances, I believe it is a responsible intervention to prevent or at least reduce the abuse of stimulant medications and opioid derivatives, especially when prescribed through telehealth platforms. It's too easy to get these medications online by giving false information to prescribers.

We must not compound the opioid crisis by supporting or working for telehealth companies that seem interested in pushing pills for profits at the expense of patient safety. Let's not lose sight of what it means to provide genuinely ethical care.

Treatment Is a Two-Way Street

*The field of mental health sometimes refers to patients
as "high functioning" or "low functioning." It's very
disparaging and demeaning to refer to patients that
way. I suppose we could apply the same terminology
to doctors to describe their level of functioning.
All doctor-patient relationships should strive to be
high-functioning — and mutually rewarding.*

I WAS READING ABOUT THE RELATIONSHIP between the pioneering psychologist Erik Erikson and the iconic painter Norman Rockwell. Erikson, who gained fame for explicating eight crucial stages of psychosocial development across the lifespan, was Rockwell's psychotherapist.

Both men lived in the idyllic Massachusetts town of Stockbridge, where Rockwell painted one of his most recognized pieces — "Stockbridge Main Street at Christmas" — depicting picturesque Main Street during the holiday season. Stockbridge Main Street was also home to the famous Austen Riggs Center, a bastion of psychoanalytic practice and long inpatient stays. Rockwell's wife was hospitalized at Austen Riggs for treatment of depression and alcohol use disorder. Rockwell, himself, fell into a deep depression, which led to a serendipitous encounter with Erikson and subsequent outpatient treatment with him.

Rockwell was fussy about his paintings — a perfectionist at heart. In a depressed state, his obsessiveness was insufferable, over-thinking his technique and questioning the quality of his artwork. Erikson pulled Rockwell out of depression and helped impart the social milieu of the 1950s into Rockwell's paintings. In audio recordings, one can hear Rockwell tell his son Tom how Erikson helped him revitalize his painting, even dispensing advice to Rockwell about how he should begin the lineage of Rockwell's celebrated "Family Tree."

One wonders whether the relationship between the two men held any meaning for Erikson. Erikson was born in Germany and emigrated to the United States at age 31. He never knew his biological father; in fact, he was initially deceived about his paternity. As Erikson wrestled with his identity, he changed his name several times, finally arriving at "Erik Erikson" and subsequently coining the term "identity crisis." According to Jane Tillman, PhD, director of the Erikson Institute, Rockwell's paintings helped suffuse Erikson's identity by enabling him to reflect on art that was quintessentially American.

Tillman's account leads me to believe that the doctor-patient relationship is, at its best, a bidirectional affair, a two-way street. Although high-functioning doctor-patient relationships are not the same in magnitude as the one between Erikson and Rockwell, who ended up good friends, they have a special give-and-take quality. My premise is that while the physician is the ostensible healer, the patient helps heal the physician, usually through subtle means uncovered after the physician reflects on a patient's visit or upon termination of the relationship.

The idea first dawned on me as a psychiatry resident. I evaluated a young woman for a relationship problem, as I briefly described in essay 4. I thought the initial session went quite well. I asked her if she would return to discuss some issues in more depth. "I'm not seeing you again," she replied. Puzzled, I asked why. "Look at your plants," she said angrily. "They're half-dead. If you can't give your plants a little TLC, how do you expect to take care of me?"

I was shocked. I had no answer. Admittedly, I never had much of a green thumb, but the patient rightly pointed out that my inaction — not watering my plants — was inexcusable. It had a profound effect on me and led to my subsequent interest in horticulture, perhaps over-compensating for a perceived failure.

As a physician, I find it much easier to give advice than receive it, which is not a surprise. If I have to see a doctor for personal reasons, the conversation starts off stilted until I tell them I am also a physician. Upon informing the doctor I am a psychiatrist, there is often an enthusiastic exchange of stories about difficult or unusual patients. Bruce Springsteen would say that physicians' collective stories are "The Ties That Bind."

My primary care physician (PCP) went to medical school and trained in my hometown of Philadelphia. He told me his wife trained in emergency medicine at the same institution where I attended medical school and did my residency (Temple University). We shared a good laugh when discussing the sundry characters known to visit emergency departments who are not really in crisis, and how difficult it was to decide whether to prioritize their medical needs or mental health needs.

The conversation quickly turned serious. The PCP informed me that at least half his patients had concomitant mental health problems that went unaddressed mainly due to time constraints (he was allotted only 15 minutes per visit). He also confessed that he didn't feel comfortable playing the role of quasi-therapist. I told him that back in the day, I was a consultation-liaison psychiatrist, and I was routinely called to assess med-surg patients. I informed the PCP he could easily brush up on psychiatry, and I recommended a couple of primers he could read, including *The Fifteen Minute Hour: Applied Psychotherapy for the Primary Care Physician*, considered a classic.

Research confirms that physicians who can emotionally engage with patients have better outcomes and higher patient satisfaction scores. When a patient perceives that their physician cares and listens to their concerns, they are more likely to comply with medical recommendations and return for follow-up visits. But there is very little research indicating that paying credence to our patients' advice and musings makes us better doctors. Can patients stimulate our personal growth, as Rockwell did for Erikson in his search for identity?

The short answer is that physicians can become better doctors by being patients. When doctors exchange the white coat for a hospital gown, they learn the importance of empathy and language and gain an appreciation for the trauma of illness and trauma of treatment. The well-known author and speaker Danielle Ofri, MD, PhD, echoed the same sentiment; she devoted an entire book to lessons she learned from her patients. One of the most important, she believes, is learning what it feels like to actually be a patient — in her case, the humiliation and helplessness she felt both during and after giving birth.

In addition to assuming the patient role, listening carefully to our patients, especially the poor and others who are disadvantaged, helps physicians grow, because learning how to overcome barriers to high-quality treatment — barriers such as poverty, poor access to care, time limits on interactions, bureaucratic red tape, and general mistrust of healthcare systems — enables physicians to adopt more personalized approaches to healthcare. Clearly, if we accept our patients as teachers, they will infuse elements of humanism in our training and practice. Patients have been known to "define our work, instantiate our values, and shape our identities," much like Rockwell aided Erikson. It is not unreasonable to expect that doctors who are exposed to diverse communities will develop strong clinical skills, become patient advocates, and contribute to a vibrant physician workforce.

It's been said that medicine is an art whose magic and creative ability reside in the interpersonal aspects of physician-patient relationships. Too often, however, medical practice has become stymied by tasks that need completing and patients that need complex services. Grinding through our day, we lose sight of what a special role we can play in patients' lives. It is only when we rediscover our passion for the practice of medicine and embrace our mission — to serve the suffering — that we realize we have the power to transform patients, and in doing so, transform ourselves.

Allegory Is a Powerful Tool in Medicine

The late comedian Joan Rivers used to say, "Can we talk?" meaning is our conversation on the same wavelength? I have found that one of the best ways to enjoin patients in crucial conversations is to use metaphors, parables and allegories. One caveat: Just be sure the message isn't lost on the patient.

I WAS LISTENING to an obscure compact disc (CD) from the equally obscure progressive rock band Caravan. The CD was titled "Blind Dog at St. Dunstans." At the end of the seventh song, "Jack and Jill," two voices can be heard amid music and barking dogs. The first voice asks, "What are those two doggies doing over there?" The second voice answers, "Well, the doggie in front is blind and his friend behind is pushing him all the way to St. Dunstans." (St. Dunstan's Hostel was founded in 1914 as a charity and rehabilitation center for British soldiers who were blinded during World War I.)

My laughter yielded to somewhat serious contemplation. How often do we use allegories, parables, and fables — stories in general — to explain complicated medical concepts to patients? Probably not often enough. But as researchers in Canada observed, "collectively, physicians' stories become ... shared awakenings to the importance of humanities in medicine."

One of the most pristine examples is the use of war as an allegory for medical intervention. Colleen Bell, PhD, a professor of political science, writes: "... metaphors of illness, patient, and physician — constituting a strategic allegory of medical intervention — have appeared as characters in the narrative of modern counterinsurgency." Bell notes that physicians have a tendency to view cancer and infectious diseases as "threats" that must be evaded. Upon successful treatment, the patient has "beaten the enemy" and "won the battle."

Plato's Allegory of the Cave has frequently been used as a teaching tool in medicine. The Allegory of the Cave describes a group of imprisoned individuals forced to live in a cave their entire lives. The prisoners can only see shadows of objects moving near a fire, but they cannot see the objects casting these shadows. The prisoners, Plato argues, are us: human beings trapped by the limitations of our senses.

Plato's cave embodies the uncertainty embedded in humans' perception of the world and the objects it contains, contrasting reality with our interpretation of it. It is a lesson in humility to know that physicians will never have perfect or complete understanding of a patient's disease. Living and working with uncertainty is why practicing medicine is considered both an art and a science.

I used many allegories with my patients. I viewed storytelling as a way to bridge the divide that separates us from human frailty. Some of my favorite allegories were based on books and movies that, in themselves, were loosely based on Plato's Cave.

For example, I treated a patient with a severe narcissistic personality disorder. He saw the world only one way: his way. I used Ray Bradbury's 1953 novel *Fahrenheit 451* to urge him to consider other viewpoints. In this famous dystopian novel, fireman Guy Montag burns books for a living, until an eccentric young neighbor forces him to reconsider his worldview.

I've treated several medical professionals for depression related to imposter syndrome (essay 15). In this context, the 1998 movie *The Truman Show* was a useful allegory. Unbeknown to Truman Burbank (Jim Carrey), he lives a faux life used purely for television entertainment. Slowly, he begins to chip away at the facade and breaks free, discovering his true identity.

When my patients with schizophrenia and bipolar disorder were in remission, many of them related to the classic 1966 French film *King of Hearts*. The inmates from the asylum literally escaped and took control over an abandoned town ravaged by war. The psychiatric patients assumed the role of shopkeepers, like "normal" people.

The most frightening and dangerous patient I ever treated was a pyromaniac. Anger and rage were at the root of his impulse disorder, and I suggested a metaphor for his anger — one that I learned from my supervisor. I told my patient that anger was like gasoline. He could use it in one of two ways: he could set the gasoline on fire with a lighted match, or he could put the gasoline in his car for extra mileage. "There is nothing wrong with being angry," I told him, "It just depends on how you use it."

My favorite allegory is the starfish story. Many of you have heard it before. In short, a little boy at the beach returns stranded starfish to the ocean. An old man asks the boy, "Do you really think you're making any difference?" The boy holds aloft one of the starfish and replies, "It makes a difference to this one," and hurls it back into the sea. The starfish allegory resonates most with patients who have given up on themselves and question why we work so diligently to save them.

I recounted to my supervisor how I planned to selectively use the starfish story. He said I had a "savior complex." "Art," he commented in the same vein as the older man to the child, "you can't save them all," reminding me that psychiatry, like other specialties, has a mortality rate – from suicide and homicide. Still, I tried.

Understanding allegories requires abstract reasoning. Therefore, children and individuals with cognitive deficits, poor comprehension, or limited English proficiency may not be appropriate candidates, because the allegory may be misunderstood or misleading.

Case in point: I was required to deliver bad news to a gay man I had been treating in psychotherapy. His comprehension was below average, and to make matters worse, AIDS was new on the horizon (circa 1983). He handed me a health department letter that read "HTLV III positive" (the term "HIV" had not yet been coined).

I thought if I explained the allegory behind Nathaniel Hawthorne's *The Scarlet Letter* — that "A" stood for adultery (among other possible meanings) and that shaming tactics do more to alienate than they do to heal — that it would affirm my patient's choice of lifestyle and lessen the blow of bad news. But the message never registered. Sensing his bewilderment, I advised my patient to discuss the lab result with his primary care physician.

I have since learned more appropriate ways to deliver bad news and how to temper my storytelling so that I can be certain to reach and join patients rather than confuse them or come across as disingenuous.

So, if you choose to use allegories in practice, make sure they are understood and paint a complete and accurate picture of the reality of the situation. After all, the dog from behind is not really guiding the dog in front!

Understanding Patients' Religious and Spiritual Beliefs Promotes Healing

Caregiving often calls us into a spiritual realm we didn't even know was possible. However, providing care in a religious context challenges the assumptions of established "good clinical practice" and raises some philosophical and treatment dilemmas for practitioners.

AN ARTICLE IN *JAMA* URGED DOCTORS to pay attention to the spiritual aspects of their calling. Spirituality was defined as "a dynamic and intrinsic aspect of humanity through which persons seek ultimate meaning, purpose, and transcendence, and experience relationship to self, family, others, community, society, nature, and the significant or sacred. Spirituality is expressed through beliefs, values, traditions, and practices."

Religious and spiritual experiences have shaped my worldview since I was a teenager. At age 13, I celebrated my bar mitzvah (the Jewish religious ritual and family celebration commemorating attaining adulthood). Later that year, I underwent an appendectomy. A priest asked my mother if he could pray for me prior to the operation. My mother did not hesitate to accept the priest's blessing. I learned at an early age that prayers for one's well-being should be welcomed regardless of the religion of the sender and recipient.

When I was a resident, I was asked to see a patient who was refusing a potentially life-saving blood transfusion. Her refusal was based on religious grounds. I asked her to consider whether God might sometimes heal through doctors. I believe physicians can legitimately claim to be a religious conduit to help guide patients' decisions about life-saving treatment.

I was once consulted about an elderly black woman experiencing somatic delusions. She complained of bizarre physical sensations that were allegedly due to rootwork, a type of voodoo specific to the African-American cultural heritage of spirituality and religion that continues to influence the health behavior of black Americans, especially in rural areas of the south. Unfortunately, I was not able to help this woman with traditional psychiatric treatment. I referred her to a healer experienced in "roots" medicine.

Whether or not physicians are religious or do not consider religion an important component of treatment, they should keep in mind that most patients value incorporating religion and spirituality in their treatment plan. In 1995, the World Health Organization declared that spirituality is an important dimension of patients' quality of life.

If physicians do not understand their patients' religious and spiritual convictions, they may be less effective in helping them. This point was well-documented in *The Healing Power of Faith: Science Explores Medicine's Last Great Frontier* by Harold G. Koenig, MD. The book focuses on the impact of traditional religious faith and practice on physical health and emotional well-being and presents concrete data showing that religion and spiritual-based beliefs are important dimensions of healing.

For example, medicine is replete with anecdotal evidence from patients claiming, "I could not have done it (quit substances, recovered from illness or surgery, beat cancer, etc.) without God's help." Religious individuals with a strong social support network often have their diseases diagnosed earlier, become actively involved in their treatments, and follow their physicians' instructions more closely than non-religious people. Religious people also cope well with stress, are less likely to be depressed and hospitalized than their nonreligious counterparts, have a stronger immune system, and live longer, according to Koenig's research.

Individuals with strong religious convictions tend to avoid unhealthy habits and lifestyles. This leads to lower rates of pulmonary disease such as emphysema and lung cancer (due to smoking), lower levels of liver disease such as cirrhosis (from alcohol use disorder), and significantly lower levels of other substance-induced disorders compared with the general population.

Many doctors believe that providing medical treatment in connection with their own spirituality improves their care. Studies suggest that over half of Americans want their doctors to speak to them about spiritual aspects of health. For many patients, faith-based medicine fosters a stronger relationship with their doctor and provides comfort in the face of chronic diseases, chronic pain and addiction. Many doctors now include faith as part of their bedside manner. At the same time, physicians must be aware of instances when patients are uncomfortable with the subject of faith and be careful not to proselytize or push their beliefs on patients.

Francisco Rosario, MD, is an internal medicine physician who has worked in New York for over 20 years. He says, "The new trend is trying to incorporate the spiritual into medicine," including praying with patients. Having faith in God (or whatever deity or spiritual essence you believe) is what makes the practice of medicine still an art despite tremendous progress in the science of medicine.

Although many physicians believe religious commitments are fine as personal values, they have segregated religion from their practice because they feel it is improper to mix the two. This type of thinking stems from the outdated doctrine that one's religious commitments should not interfere with standard medical care and that comingling personal beliefs with medical practice is not what medical authorities or patients expect of physicians. Increasingly, however, physicians find that ethos unsatisfying spiritually and intellectually. They have come to recognize that health and well-being are optimized by combining the best that science and religion offer.

There's a classic "Gates of Heaven" joke about a man who drowned that I've sometimes told to skeptical colleagues and patients (obviously, jokes aren't right for everyone). The joke goes like this:

A fellow was stuck on his rooftop in a flood. He was praying to God for help. Soon a man in a rowboat came by, and the fellow shouted to the man on the roof, "Jump in; I can save you." The stranded fellow shouted back, "No, it's OK, I'm praying to God, and he is going to save me." So, the rowboat went on.

221

Then a motorboat came by. "The fellow in the motorboat shouted, "Jump in; I can save you." To this, the stranded man said, "No thanks, I'm praying to God, and he is going to save me. I have faith." So, the motorboat went on.

Then a helicopter came by, and the pilot shouted down, "Grab this rope, and I will lift you to safety." To this, the stranded man again replied, "No thanks, I'm praying to God, and he is going to save me. I have faith." So, the helicopter reluctantly flew away.

Soon the water rose above the rooftop, and the man drowned. He went to heaven. He finally got his chance to discuss this whole situation with God, at which point the man exclaimed, "I had faith in you, but you didn't save me. You let me drown. I don't understand why!" God replied to this, "I sent you a rowboat, a motorboat, and a helicopter. What more did you expect?"

ESSAY 60

What Does It Mean When We Say Someone Has Died After a Long Illness?

*Readers can't help but notice my references to, and
passion for, rock and roll music. When rock icon
David Crosby died "after a long illness" yet seemed
perfectly fine on the day of his death, it left many
of his admirers perplexed, including yours truly. I
discovered the answer to the question posed in the
title of this essay through personal introspection.*

ONE OF MY DOCTORS and two of my cherished mentors (essays 37
and 38) died within the past several years, each "after a long illness,"
according to their obituaries. Rock legend David Crosby (The Byrds
and Crosby, Stills, Nash & Young) died "after a long illness," as
reported by his wife, Jan Dance.

David Crosby's co-musicians were perplexed that his widow
would attribute his death to a long illness. Crosby certainly had his
share of health concerns — substance use, hepatitis C, liver trans-
plant, cardiac catheterization, and diabetes — and he frequently
joked about his death, planning his funeral in advance. However,
in his final days, Crosby's new bandmates observed him "writing,
playing [and] singing his ass off." The day he died, Crosby "seemed
practically giddy with all of it," working on a new album and planning a tour. At 81, his vocal ability remained top-notch, even if
arthritis made playing the guitar difficult. The fact is, David Crosby's
final decade of life was his most vibrant, releasing five studio albums.
His sudden death was understandably puzzling.

As a psychiatrist, I am accustomed to reading that someone
has died after a long illness. I know that in many cases, the illness

is depressive in nature, and the individual has died by suicide. The "long illness" is sometimes a euphemism for suicide, a word we struggle to say out loud. I can certainly understand why families would want to keep suicide a secret, given the stigma attached to it and the stigma that continues to surround mental illness in general. But unless we confront the epidemic of suicide, the problem will continue to fester, and we'll never be able to break through the cloud of silence.

Perhaps we are more at ease discussing death due to medical illnesses than death due to mental illnesses, Crosby's death notwithstanding. Even conditions once dreaded and believed to be horrifying and incurable, such as cancer and HIV/AIDS, are discussed openly — advertising their treatment on television to millions with catchy, upbeat melodies in the background (see essay 54). So, why do family members still prefer the term "after a long illness" as a code for conditions that result in death? Crosby's guitar player commented: "He was a weakened guy from many different preexisting conditions, and everyone knew it..." Why not say what those conditions are?

The answer is: Respect and privacy trump the need to know. However well-intentioned I may think it is to disseminate information about someone's cause of death, the family's interests in the matter override mine. Crosby's fans were curious to know more about his death, but his wife had the final say, as it should be. (Ironically, her refusal to go into detail led people to probe her background.)

I was reminded of the sanctity of death in an account by Ashley Judd to *The New York Times* about her mother, Naomi, that I referenced in essay 45. You may recall that the iconic country singer Naomi Judd died by suicide in April 2022. Several months later, her daughter Ashley penned a guest essay in *The New York Times* about her family's efforts to keep police reports related to the suicide private, including photographs and body cam footage. Judd wrote: "Though I acknowledge the need for law enforcement to investigate a sudden violent death by suicide, there is absolutely no compelling public interest in the case of my mother to justify releasing the videos, images, and family interviews that were done in the course of that investigation."

At the urging of the Judd family, Tennessee Senator Jack Johnson introduced legislation to make death investigation records private when the death is not the result of a crime. Judd remarked: "The raw details [of death] are used only to feed a craven gossip economy, and as we cannot count on basic human decency, we need laws that will compel that restraint." A catch-22 is that public disclosure of the nature of the death may be required to determine whether it is or is not the result of a crime, but such instances are rare.

Judd pointed out that a big problem for law enforcement personnel is that they are not adequately trained to respond to and investigate trauma-related cases. They employ outdated interview procedures and methods of interacting with family members who are in shock and grieving. Not only are families at their most vulnerable following the acute death of a loved one, but in Judd's case, she felt "cornered and powerless" when interrogated by the police, "stripped of any sensitive boundary," as though she were a suspect. Ashley Judd had to re-enter trauma-focused psychotherapy to deal with the events.

In addition, Judd wrote that her family felt "deep compassion" for Vanessa Bryant, the wife of NBA star Kobe Bryant who was killed along with his daughter and other passengers in a 2020 helicopter crash. Like the Judd family (and other families), Bryant had to endure the release of details surrounding the deaths. Families and their memories of deceased relatives deserve respect. To say that someone has died after a long illness, regardless of the specific cause of death, gives them that respect.

Regrettably, attempts to describe cryptic deaths are frequently inaccurate or maligned. One of my doctors did indeed die "after a long illness." He was my neurosurgeon, and he died tragically by suicide (see essay 45). When I clicked on his "link" to an affiliated hospital's website a week later, I received an error message: "Page not found." Worse yet, Queen Elizabeth's death was attributed to "old age," as meager, and some would say ageist, as describing an elderly person's death as "natural causes" or "failure to thrive." The latter term originated in the pediatric world and has now migrated to geriatrics and might best be avoided.

I've kidded my family about what to write in my obituary and on my gravestone and how to divide my possessions when my time comes. In the final analysis, however, people should be remembered for how they lived, not for how they died, and certainly not for the private details of how they may have suffered.

Don't Let Vindictiveness Creep into Medicine Like It Has in Politics

The border crossing of migrants into the United States and their subsequent bussing to faraway destinations has parallels in medicine.

THE CALLOUS AND INHUMANE DISLOCATION of migrants perpetrated by governors of the states of Florida and Texas reminded me of an equally disdainful and appalling tactic utilized by healthcare workers since the 1960s: "Greyhound therapy."

Greyhound therapy refers to attempts by healthcare workers and administrators to remove undesirable patients from emergency rooms, hospitals, and other types of facilities by providing them one-way tickets on a Greyhound Lines bus to another far-away location, hoping they will never return. Some of the patients are troublemakers and rabble-rousers known to frequent emergency departments, but the majority are destitute, homeless, or mentally ill — or all three — and deserve our compassion.

Greyhound therapy is still in play in certain medical and mental-health circles. Between 2013 and 2018, a state-run psychiatric hospital in Nevada routinely bused patients to places they had never been or had no ties to, providing only a few days of food rations and medication for the trip. A class-action lawsuit was filed against the hospital on behalf of approximately 1,500 patients who were cast off, and a Las Vegas jury returned a unanimous verdict in favor of the patients, awarding each person $250,000 for the hospital's egregious treatment.

A far more common but no less derisive practice is patient "dumping" — discharging uninsured and undesirable patients to the street or transferring them to another facility. Patient dumping was — and still is — such a huge problem that it literally has required an act of Congress to stop it: the federal anti-dumping law passed in 1986 known as the Emergency Medical Treatment and Active Labor Act (EMTALA).

Under EMTALA, patients must be medically screened and stabilized prior to discharge or transfer. If a hospital is unable to stabilize a patient given its resources, or if the patient requests, a transfer may be made with the consent of the receiving hospital.

Greyhound therapy, dumping, and the busing of migrant workers have their roots in the "Freedom Riders." Freedom Riders were civil rights activists who rode interstate buses into segregated southern states in 1961 to challenge Jim Crow laws that remained in force despite Supreme Court decisions that outlawed segregation in schools and public buses and depots.

To embarrass Northern liberals and humiliate black people, southern White Citizens Councils and other groups countered the Freedom Riders. "Reverse Freedom Riders" issued black people one-way tickets to northern cities with false promises of jobs, housing, and better lives. The Kennedy administration received mail from leaders in the targeted states asking the federal government to intervene in the cruel trafficking of people of color.

The past behavior of bigots is remarkably similar to the current behavior of the governors of Florida and Texas. As one columnist observed, the two governors simply followed an old playbook by shipping the migrants north. The governors were not clever. They were racist. At least officials in Arizona coordinated their efforts to relocate migrants.

The recent display of vindictiveness shown by the governors cannot be attributed to implicit bias. Implicit bias originates in prejudices that unknowingly influence how people are treated, especially minorities. There is nothing unknowing or unconscious in the minds of those who orchestrate and approve the trafficking of vulnerable populations.

Exploiting people's misery for political gain is shameful and no more acceptable than sending patients on dead-end journeys. JFK characterized the Reverse Freedom Riders as "a rather cheap shot." He envisioned government contractors would treat their employees without regard to their race, creed, color, or national origin. Shouldn't the same hold true for health professionals?

The notion of equal medical treatment dates back to Hippocrates. He stated: "Into whatever homes I go, I will enter them for the benefit of the sick ... whether they are free men or slaves." In many U.S. medical schools, it has become customary for incoming medical students to write and recite their own versions of the Hippocratic Oath. Many of the variants include language that specifically prohibits discrimination or bias in the practice of medicine.

I have often wondered about the state of mind of healthcare providers who approve of one-way travel as a solution to homelessness, drug addiction, and mental illness. Health officials in Nevada strung together a thin veil of excuses, ranging from denial to arguing that they were sending patients directly to family members and other mental health facilities — possibly true in a few cases but utterly false in a majority of them. Clearly, there was a blatant disregard for human rights fueled by prejudice and stigma against the mentally ill.

Nevada is not alone in its brazen treatment of psychiatric patients, nor do southern states own the exclusive rights to export its citizens. New York City secretly sends the homeless to Hawaii and other states. Only in rare instances does travel therapy aim to be genuinely therapeutic.

For example, Hawaii has attempted to reunite homeless people with relatives on the mainland, so-called airplane therapy. But due to the high cost of running such a program and the fact that approximately one-third of Hawaii's population is transient or from out of state, the number of needy people who actually benefit is very small.

Vindictive politics, whether inside the Capitol or the hospital C-suite, should never take precedence over people. Anyone — politician, provider, or health care administrator — who uses human beings as pawns for leverage or personal gain, or displaces or disrupts their medical treatment for prejudiced reasons, should be guided through serious self-reflection around how racism has entered their lives and, more importantly, affected the lives of innocent and disadvantaged patients.

Leaders and caregivers must never forget the welcoming inscription engraved on the base of the Statue of Liberty: "give me your tired your poor" and especially the words that follow: "Send these, the homeless, tempest-tost to me." Migrants, like many of our patients, are overwhelmed by life's circumstances. We are, and always have been, a nation that opens its arms to vulnerable people rather than consigns them to a destination far worse than where their journey began.

Practice Management

I Retired After Being Punished for Speaking Out. Now I Can Speak My Mind

If you feel betrayed by your employer or unsupported by your coworkers, you should be prepared to have difficult conversations with those in charge — or consider leaving for a better job.

I WORKED 40 YEARS AS an employed clinician, but I always feared losing my job. There were many reasons to be scared: mergers, acquisitions, downsizing, and potential conflicts with new bosses, to name a few. However, the primary reason I feared losing my job was for speaking my mind.

Existing in a constant state of anxiety due to job insecurity is a terrible way to live. But, as the sole earner for a family of four children and a spouse, I felt I could not afford to take any chances, and the greatest risk I perceived was voicing my opinion about something negative at work. Let's face it: Nobody likes a whiner or a whistleblower. The problem is, the less you say, the more you enable others to define your voice and your identity.

Had I owned my practice rather than worked for healthcare organizations all my life, things might have been different. Nowadays, however, more than 50% of physicians are employed, so my experience is quite relevant. I worked at academic medical centers and pharmaceutical and health insurance companies. Clinicians working in the industry are considerably outnumbered by the "suits" and must conform to business values that may clash with patient care values.

Sometimes, for example, business dictates that the truth be hidden, like refraining from publishing the outcomes of negative clinical trials. Physicians working in-house as medical directors for large corporations also walk a fine line when organizational demands intrude on their obligations to individual employees. Companies may try to downplay physicians' opinions that employees' illnesses are work-related.

When I was 41, I was approached by the CEO of a psychiatric hospital where I was CMO. The hospital was about to default on a substantial loan that could bankrupt the hospital and the CEO wanted me to listen in on a telephone conversation between the CEO, the CFO, and the bank loan officer. The CEO fabricated an excuse for why the hospital was in default, and he promised to satisfy the payment if the loan officer granted him a two-week extension. The loan officer agreed.

The CEO and CFO smiled smugly and chuckled after the call, leaving me tangled in their web of lies. Somehow, they made the payment, but soon after, the hospital was again on the brink of bankruptcy. It was acquired by another healthcare system, proving the adage that you can call yourself an "acquired health care company" and be correct half of the time. I saw the handwriting on the wall after that call and changed jobs before the acquisition.

I've felt muzzled throughout my career due to the fear that my opinions might not sit well with individuals who rank above me in the organization.

Many well-intentioned bloggers have shared their tips for speaking your mind at work. They tend to frame the issue in terms of courage rather than fear. They ask, "What's the most courageous act you ever did at work?" Employees' responses are remarkably consistent, such as, "I stood up to my boss," "I shared truthful information no one wanted to hear," and "I argued an unpopular point of view."

However, none of their answers speak to the nuanced practice of a physician.

In the world of medicine, opinions can be dangerous and politicized. Expressing a controversial opinion can damage your reputation; stating a belief that contradicts the medical establishment can leave you vulnerable; voicing your opinion at the wrong time can make you appear foolish. The axiom attributed to Abraham

Lincoln goes: "Better to remain silent and be thought a fool than to speak and remove all doubt." One can easily see how this mantra may inhibit physicians in their practice of medicine.

My first week into a job with a renowned pharmaceutical company, I challenged the senior vice president (a physician) regarding the feasibility of conducting a clinical trial on depression. I was in favor of the trial, but the senior vice president was not inclined to fund it. I argued my rationale to them, and the next thing I knew my boss was advising me to back off. He said he had just saved my hide, as the senior vice president was disposed to firing me — simply for speaking my mind in opposition.

Another time, while working in the health insurance industry, I outlined a comprehensive plan to manage mental health benefits for the company's insureds. I suggested that the company carve in mental health benefits rather than carve them out, as was the prevalent arrangement at that time and still is today. A couple of weeks later, the CMO told me he was eliminating mental health benefits, a euphemism for eliminating my job rather than the benefits per se. The back-to-back blows I suffered while working in the industry further silenced me and curtailed any aspiration for a position in the C-suite.

I retired when I reached full retirement age (as defined by the Social Security Administration) and when my return on lifetime investments provided sufficient income. To help pass the time, I began consulting from home. My consulting business has grown. But the important thing is I feel I have nothing to lose by speaking my mind, because if a client were to drop me today, I would still be financially independent. My clients seem to like me and appreciate my openness, directness, and honesty. My "retirement" has allowed me to speak my voice — ironically, at a time when I was not expecting to work anymore.

If your employer would fire you because you voiced an unpopular opinion, you shouldn't be working there.

Is Fear of Retaliation Silencing Doctors?

We must speak out on issues impacting the well-being of our patients and ourselves. At the same time, we must follow corporate policies (where they exist) that require approval to publicly discuss or publish our opinions. When these two obligations clash, which path will you follow?

LIKE MANY BABY BOOMERS who grew up in the Vietnam War era and protested it on college campuses, I came to resent authority and relish free speech. So, I was curious to read that a Mayo Clinic doctor was fired for publishing a book that included criticism of Mayo's handling of the COVID-19 crisis. Apparently, the physician failed to follow Mayo's publication policy, which required Mayo officials to review the book prior to publication.

I also read about a pediatrician working as a health official in Tennessee who was fired after she campaigned to get teens vaccinated for COVID-19. (Tennesseans lagged behind much of the nation in COVID-19 vaccination rates.)

Many other doctors have been fired or threatened termination from their jobs for speaking out against policies and practices that put patients at risk, and their concerns were not merely COVID-19 related. Judging by the experience of those physicians and the Mayo doctor, it appears that speaking out, especially about controversial issues, can result in career suicide. But none of this is new.

In 1998, a survey of 465 emergency physicians revealed that approximately 25% felt their jobs were threatened by voicing quality of care or equitable compensation concerns. A 2013 survey confirmed that emergency physicians continue to experience anxiety about job security, and physicians in other specialties fear they may lose their jobs after speaking out about unsafe conditions. To silence them, a prominent New York health system emailed staff members telling them that if they talk to the media without permission, they "will be subject to disciplinary action, including termination."

Several colleagues have confided in me that they have worked for companies they believe are unsafe or unethical, yet they hesitate to speak out because of the prospect of losing their jobs. One individual told me he "was in the throes of a difficult situation," and was trying to navigate through it with the aid of a labor attorney. What could be so terrible, I thought, that my colleague had to enlist an attorney to help him resolve his situation? Then I flashed back to a time in my own career when I assumed the role of chief medical officer of a hospital. On my first day at work, the former CMO unceremoniously appeared at my doorway and shouted, "You're working for snakes." He was correct (see the preceding essay). I left that job in less than two years. And my colleague ended up relocating to take a job more in line with his values.

In present day, some highly vocal and opinionated doctors have resorted to social media to air their grievances. They really put their jobs on the line, however. Rule number one for physicians using social media to protest a cause is that they should think of the internet as the world's elevator: Passengers along for the ride listen to the conversation and never forget.

Internet transgressions are not necessarily blatant. For example, as discussed in essay 28, a credible group of researchers published an article examining the social media habits of surgical residents with the intent to "empower surgeons" by making them aware of how their posts on Facebook, Twitter, and Instagram may affect patient and public perceptions. However, the result backfired. The young surgeons were not empowered at all. Rather, they felt targeted and violated (the researchers had never obtained permission to access their online accounts) and the resulting backlash forced the researchers to retract their article and the journal editors to issue an apology.

Yet, the idea of empowering physicians is gaining traction because doctors are increasingly becoming employees trapped in systems that are not working for them or for the benefit of their patients. Physicians continue to report significant concerns regarding their ability to speak out about the quality of care and financial incentives that favor the bottom lines of healthcare systems over the safety of patients. Doctors who choose to speak their mind increasingly feel they will be ignored, censored, or fired, often without due process.

Of course, there's an important distinction between a doctor speaking out against unfair policies or in the interest of a patient, and those who are breaking a law or putting patients at risk. For example, health providers have been fired or reprimanded by state medical licensing boards for posting content that identifies patients, which is a clear HIPAA violation. Others have lost their jobs for espousing radical or unfounded beliefs and for making racist comments.

But the line between good and bad, right and wrong, isn't always so clear. The question then becomes, how can doctors be given the space to speak out in a manner that promotes autonomy and protects patient safety while ensuring they aren't causing harm? Until healthcare systems recognize and change those policies that unjustly quiet physicians, it falls on doctors to work within the bounds of the system to make their voices heard.

A good rule of thumb is that if a policy harms or has the potential to injure patients, the physician should speak out and "resist and even refuse to carry it out," according to the late medical ethicist Edmund Pellegrino, MD. To comply with bad medical practices is a violation of the covenant between the doctor and the patient. Physicians must have the fortitude, however, to leave their jobs when it becomes apparent that their concerns are disregarded by institutions or that they might be censored for advocating for patients.

Moreover, prior to accepting a job, physicians should become aware of their institution's policies regarding publishing (op-eds, articles, books, etc.) and posting on social media. I thoroughly enjoyed working in industry the latter half of my career, yet I felt gagged by some companies' publication policies that required pre-clearance, as in the case of the Mayo Clinic. Depending on my employer's policies,

I either refrained from publishing or I published with a disclaimer, such as: "The author's opinions are his own and not necessarily those of [the company, institution, professional organization, etc.]."

As much as I dislike the idea of censoring physicians, I recognize there are limits to free speech. At least I had the autonomy to accept or not accept a job offer. It can't be called censorship when you voluntarily agree to abide by the rules of an organization and then are fired for knowingly breaking those rules.

Professional Courtesy Means Being a "Doctor's Doctor"

If we don't make our colleagues' health a priority and provide them rapid assessment and treatment, there will be very few healthy doctors left to treat the public.

I HAD AN EMAIL EXCHANGE with a friend and psychiatric colleague, Michael Myers, MD, on the topic of professional courtesy. I wrote about professional courtesy in essay 44. That op-ed stirred considerable controversy, so much so that readers' comments turned ugly and unprofessional (refer to essays 2 and 3) and the commenting section on the host website was closed. It seems my op-ed struck a raw nerve primarily among millennials, many of whom were unfamiliar with the concept of professional courtesy and strongly objected to it once it became clear to them that I expected preferential treatment from other physicians for me or my family members — treatment in the form of discounted fees or quick appointments, or both. Readers considered me "privileged" and "entitled."

An article about Myers characterized him as a "doctor's doctor" because he specializes in treating physicians and their families. He noted that the culture of medicine surrounding the treatment of physicians with mental illness and substance use disorders has significantly improved in the past several decades. But physicians suffering from mental disorders are still shunned and marginalized by physicians in mainstream medicine, especially those in positions of leadership and authority, who continue to buy into the myth that if a physician or medical trainee becomes psychiatrically ill, he or she may not be fit to practice medicine, or may not have been cut out for it.

Although mental health stigma has lessened, it persists, and there is a great need for psychiatrists — indeed, for all physicians — to be on guard and available for their colleagues in times of need. Helping physicians recover from mental illness or substance use disorders is rewarding for the individual, the practitioner, and the profession. I regret that I never had a chance to explain this to readers who impugned my essay.

I was never given a second chance to tell them how unfair it is that our mentally burdened colleagues tend to be judged by institutional and archaic rules of medicine. I never had the opportunity to remind them that Sir Francis Peabody famously said: "One of the essential qualities of the clinician is interest in humanity, for the secret of the care of the patient is in caring for the patient." And I wasn't able to appeal to their reasoning by informing them that groomers at PetSmart have more autonomy to book longer appointments for their pets than physicians do for their patients.

I felt vindicated when I read Myers' comment that he "grew up in the era of what was called 'professional courtesy' – the idea that as fellow professionals, we look after our own. It's very gratifying work. You can help so many people who are in turn helping others get well." When Myers and I conducted a workshop at the annual meeting of the American Psychiatric Association (in 2016) for physicians with practice-related PTSD (essay 25), it generated tremendous interest and a standing-room-only crowd.

Many physicians spoke candidly about their personal experiences with trauma in the course of practicing — either first-hand or witnessed traumatic experiences — and one psychiatrist broke down in tears while telling her story (refer to essay 26). We asked her to stay afterward to share more of her experience. She had been traumatized by a recent divorce and fell victim to vicarious trauma while treating patients at a Veterans Affairs hospital. We gave her the names of professionals in her area she could contact for further help and possible psychiatric treatment. She deeply appreciated our concern and that we were willing to spend extra time with her. I have stayed in touch with this doctor over the years. She is doing quite well; to ease the pain of her trauma, she left practice for a non-clinical career.

In my email exchange with Myers, he wrote: "There is a middle ground [to professional courtesy]. I think that we can still offer [it] to each other without actually accepting the new patient ourselves. I've done this a lot over the years. I call the colleague back ASAP but certainly by the end of the day, explain my situation, then offer the names of one or two colleagues whom I highly recommend who I think would see the colleague (or their family member). If the caller demurs, then I offer to call the folks myself. Obviously, this is time-consuming but I've found that simply taking the referral seriously and trying to assist makes the colleague feel respected and heard."

"Years ago," he continued, "when I was practicing in Vancouver, I was treating a physician for severe depression, but she also had horrendous migraines. I called one of our local headache specialists, a neurologist, who at that time had a waiting list for a year (remember, this is Canada). He took my call, listened for a minute or two, and said, 'Have her contact my receptionist. I'll see her tomorrow night at 7 p.m. If we can't help each other in our hour of need, then medicine is really f***ed.' I was so grateful. When I called my patient and told her about the appointment, she sobbed with relief."

Whether the diagnosis is depression, PTSD, substance use disorder, or some other mental health condition, many of our peers are like the two physician patients described herein: filled with pent-up emotion, ready to burst at the seams, and incredibly appreciative of colleagues going the extra mile to ensure their well-being. Call it professional courtesy or simply old-fashioned medicine — our colleagues deserve no less. Let's heed Peabody's call to the basics of our humanity and restore humility and decency in medicine. We should all aspire to be a "doctor's doctor."

A Message to Physician Job Recruiters: First Impressions Count

Human resource professionals represent the face of a company. If they are unfriendly, disorganized, or unaware of the details of the job, take that as a sign the company (and job) may not be the right one for you.

MORE THAN HALF OF ALL PHYSICIANS in the United States are employed by healthcare organizations, and the numbers have been trending upward. Recruiters who work for health systems are tasked with finding the best physicians available, and their roles have become more important than ever. In-house job recruiters and recruiters contracted with health systems represent the face of the organization. They are often the first contact for physicians in a busy and competitive marketplace, where demand for skilled physicians far outstrips supply in many areas, which gives physicians considerable leverage in selecting a job.

Healthcare recruiters must realize the importance of their initial interactions with job candidates. You would think they do, but my experience suggests otherwise. In 2022, I completed an online job application for a position with a prominent healthcare system in my area. Two days after I applied for the job, I received an email from a human resources (HR) department recruiter asking me about my availability to discuss the position. Several days after supplying the information, I received a second email from a different recruiter in the HR department, again requesting my availability.

Finally, when we connected, the recruiter told me that she was the one who was "on point" for the position — not her colleague who had sent me the initial email. In our conversation, it became quite clear that the recruiter knew very little about the position, especially the clinical responsibilities. When I asked if there were opportunities at the executive (non-clinical) level, she was uncertain and advised me to continue to search their website. The recruiter could not forward my CV internally because she did not know her counterpart who handled executive positions, nor was she inclined to seek out someone I could speak with and attempt a warm transfer of the phone call.

I realize this person is only one individual and is not necessarily representative of the culture of the organization. But first impressions count a lot. Contrast this encounter with one I had years ago when I applied for a job in the health insurance sector, one that required relocation. Not only was the recruiter extremely knowledgeable — he actually helped develop and write the job description — he handled all the minutiae of the hiring process with aplomb and reassurance. After all, relocating to a new city with a spouse and family is never an easy decision.

The recruiter imbued me with optimism and positivity about the role and the opportunity (a vice president position); he made it difficult for me to resist. He sold me on the job, convincing me it was the right move for my family and me, which it was at that time. The recruiter stayed in touch after I was hired, and we became friends — as did our spouses and children — and today, he leads the executive recruitment function for one of the largest hospital companies in the United States.

Eventually, I left the insurance company to take a job in big pharma. The hiring process there was equally impressive and seamless, including rigorous interviews, shadowing an employee, and a pre-employment physical examination for my benefit, all of which demonstrated that the company considered me a potential asset and really cared about my welfare.

I've always considered the HR department, its job recruiters, and the onboarding process — whether it was well organized or haphazard — a portent of the quality and integrity of the company. Recruiters that I've found most helpful and qualified possessed the following qualities: understanding the position responsibilities and requirements; quickly getting to the essence of a candidate's professional experience; assessing the candidate's expectations, needs, and wants; identifying and summarizing the most compelling aspects of a job opportunity; moving candidates efficiently through the pipeline; and conveying to the hiring manager what makes each candidate uniquely suited for the job.

If recruiters sound like they don't know what they're talking about, candidates may not trust them or may form a negative impression about the job or the organization. Healthcare organizations cannot afford to let talented physicians slip through their fingers because they are turned off by recruiters who underwhelm or make rookie mistakes. Health systems must invest in their HR departments, provide extensive training to personnel responsible for recruiting physicians, and monitor recruiters' performance and outcomes.

I vividly recall the car dealership where I bought my first luxury car. During my initial visit — and all subsequent visits — I encountered the same pleasant woman every time I entered the building. Her title was Director of First Impressions. Healthcare organizations should take heed.

Is It Time to Explore Alternative and Encore Careers in Medicine?

It's never too late to redo your career if you're dissatisfied with practice. Non-clinical jobs in medicine are abundant, as are other jobs distanced from clinical pursuits. Part-time working is exploding. Find a job that really matters to you.

I'M READING A LOT MORE STORIES about doctors leaving medicine for good. An internal medicine physician wants to spend more time with her children. A primary care physician wants to attend to his mentally handicapped adult son. A surgeon needs to escape a "toxic" workplace. A doctor has no avenue of appeal after he is unfairly reported to the National Practitioner Data Bank. A family medicine physician retires prematurely because practicing medicine has lost its luster and become a grind. A physician recollects, "The thing about primary care is 'poop rolls downhill,' and I'm absolutely glad I'm out of it."

The stories and reasons for leaving go on and on, but one theme most stories have in common is the realization that physicians no longer control their professional destiny — it's in the hands of attorneys, corporate CEOs, government officials, and the like. Physicians have committed their lives, careers, and income to employers they must tolerate and who insist that they practice medicine only in the way that produces the greatest income for the organization.

To be sure, the coronavirus pandemic hastened the exodus of physicians from practice. But the firestorm was ignited long before COVID-19 arrived on the scene, when, at baseline, physicians were overworked, underpaid, bogged down, second-guessed, litigated, and burned out beyond belief. The pandemic simply brought the cauldron to a boiling point.

In a perverse way, some physicians have laid the blame for this misfortune at their own doorstep. On the one hand, it is recognized that physicians fought tirelessly on the COVID-19 frontlines and were casualties of a broken healthcare system. At the same time, however, the medical profession has been denigrated by its own kind who do not consider their peers "heroes," reasoning that responding heroically to an emergency is to be expected. Nonsense! Is "heroic" not the right adjective to describe the courageous behavior of healthcare professionals during a pandemic? Why shouldn't doctors consider themselves health heroes, battling forces seen and unseen pre-COVID, during COVID, and in the pandemic's wake?

To add insult to injury, medical decision-making has been taken away from us. Nowadays, with preauthorization requirements (essay 52), it's difficult just to get patients to first base. Requested medications and procedures go through bottom-line oriented algorithms and lesser trained individuals only to land squarely back in our laps, forcing a change in treatment plans or an appeal of the denial of care. COVID-related decisions that should have been medically based — masking, vaccinating, quarantining, gathering, etc. — slipped through our grasp and into the firm hands of politicians and science naysayers.

Where does that leave physicians relative to their practice autonomy? Whatever happened to the sheer joy of practicing medicine: rendering care to patients unencumbered by third parties; enthusiastically imparting pearls of wisdom to trainees eager to learn; and providing sage advice and guidance to the next generation of physicians?

Until medicine crumbles and the public demands that doctors be placed back in charge, I don't see a way out of this mess except to explore alternative and "encore careers." The latter choice simply means that doctors will end up doing something they love but have delayed doing for the sake of medical practice. They will undertake new and meaningful vocations that traditionally played out later in their careers, only the timeline is now accelerated.

This could be good news! I wrote about encore careers in essays 18 and 19. The possibilities are endless: Physicians have turned to careers in music, art, literature, coffee roasting, wine making, and many other satisfying endeavors.

A slew of options exists for physicians who wish to leave practice but stay involved in the medical profession. Chief among them are careers in the pharmaceutical and health insurance industries. I have discouraged physicians from the latter because most of those jobs have limited career potential, and some of the actions of physicians conducting utilization review have left a stain on the practice of medicine.

Plum jobs in the pharmaceutical industry are becoming more competitive. Fortunately, there is a vast array of positions to choose from among multiple therapeutic and functional areas, such as pharmacovigilance, medical affairs, R&D, and field work. Working in the field as a medical liaison is a good way to break into the industry. Popular non-pharmaceutical jobs include medical writing and editing, consulting, and disability claims file reviews. A book by Sylvie Stacy, MD, MPH, *50 Nonclinical Careers for Physicians*, explores these and other possibilities in greater detail.

Practicing medicine was once an ideal. Practicing medicine was once a coveted profession. Practicing was once enjoyable. I'm confident that disenfranchised physicians can find something more rewarding than clinical work (abuse). Now is the time to build back better until — and if — the real thing comes along again.

Artificial Intelligence is Worse than the Old Boss

Artificial intelligence (AI) offers an unprecedented opportunity to augment what physicians can do: diagnose and treat diseases with ever greater accuracy and efficiency. However, systems built around AI are only as intelligent — and ethical — as the people who design them. Proper safeguards are required to protect against biases, errors, and patient harm.

IT SEEMS THAT EACH POSITIVE STORY I read about the benefits of artificial intelligence (AI) is countered by a negative story.

One internal medicine physician writes: "Someday, with enough computing power and artificial intelligence, we may be able to have systems that can do some basic medical advice and education about health care that could end up saving doctors a lot of time and helping patients get to a better state of health."

However, another physician observes that although AI can make medicine more efficient — particularly AI-based on computer algorithms — it can also generate "false flags" that lead to erroneous conclusions if doctors are too dependent upon technology and rely solely on system conclusions. "After all," the physician reasons, "even though it's a computer algorithm, it was devised by a human."

It's noteworthy that Geoffrey Hinton, considered the "Godfather of Artificial Intelligence" quit Google, warning of the dangers of AI. The neural network pioneer told *The New York Times* (May 1, 2023) that chatbots could be "quite scary," and he cautioned they could be exploited by "bad actors" (see essay 73).

Likewise, Samuel Altman, the head of OpenAI, the artificial intelligence company that makes ChatGPT — a free chatbot tool that answers medical and other types of questions with convincingly human-like responses — testified before Congress (May 16, 2023) that government regulation "will be critical to mitigate the risks of increasingly powerful" AI systems.

Prescription drug monitoring programs (PDMPs) are a prime example of AI gone awry, particularly the algorithmic backbone of some of these systems. PDMPs are electronic databases that track controlled substance prescriptions in individual states. In many instances, PDMPs can be integrated into electronic health record systems, permitting physicians to delegate PDMP access to advanced level providers in their office.

PDMPs are designed to monitor changes in prescribing behaviors and detect patients' use of multiple healthcare prescribers, but because they cannot capture the nuances of clinical encounters, even the CDC has admitted that PDMPs have shortcomings and "mixed" findings. The CDC often refers to PDMPs as a "promise" rather than a real fix that prevents doctors from making aberrant prescribing decisions.

Addiction specialist Maia Szalavitz has chronicled nightmarish stories of patients denied necessary pain medication due to unintelligent systems based on flawed algorithms that lead physicians to believe patients are doctor shopping or somehow at risk of becoming addicted. Women and racial minorities are disproportionately impacted by these systems, as are patients with cancer and mental disorders, despite their use of controlled substances at a rate no higher than would normally be expected to treat debilitating pain or psychiatric symptoms, respectively.

A major drawback of AI systems is their failure to account for known risk factors for addiction, such as adverse childhood experiences and mental illnesses. PDMPs may actually reinforce historical discrimination and make the opioid crisis worse by recapitulating inequalities associated with race, class, and gender and targeting patients with legitimate needs, forcing them to obtain controlled substances surreptitiously or go without them.

This all amounts to the withholding of essential pain medications and other controlled substances — especially those intended to improve mental health and well-being — from individuals who truly need them, either because doctors won't write the prescriptions once they've checked the PDMP database, or pharmacists won't fill the prescriptions.

New research shows that nearly half of medical clinics in the United States now refuse to see new patients who require opioids. I've read many accounts of the harm and humiliation created by PDMPs, even when the patients are healthcare providers themselves (their relatively high rates of addiction notwithstanding). Here are just a few examples:

A physician who specializes in informatics undergoes a complicated tooth extraction. Her pain needs to be managed by a second, more powerful, analgesic medication. Despite having a proper prescription, the pharmacist refuses to fill the medication until he personally verifies it with the patient's PCP. The physician feels embarrassed by shoppers who stare at her in line, causing her to feel like a drug addict.

A physician assistant requires extensive abdominal surgery. Her surgeon has devised a "fast-track" post-operative program in which he uses only acetaminophen for pain control. The woman, who has no history of substance use disorder, asks for a short course of opiate medication instead. The surgeon is unwavering in his adherence to the program, and the woman is coerced into seeking surgery elsewhere.

A psychiatrist has an established diagnosis of ADHD. He has been prescribed methylphenidate (Ritalin) for over 30 years, usually filled at his local pharmacy. On one occasion he decides to have the prescription filled at a pharmacy close to where he works. The pharmacist interrogates the psychiatrist in front of customers, refuses to fill the prescription, and insists that the psychiatrist have it filled at his local pharmacy.

Companies that market AI systems tell providers that computer analyses are not intended to be the sole determinants of a patient's risk of addiction. Still, pharmacists have the "right" to fill a prescription — or not. They can rely on the output of PDMPs and, in addition, interject their own biases and prejudices to deny patients much-needed medication (some states allow pharmacists the absolute right to refuse to provide services). Patients lose when prescribing physicians defer to unwilling pharmacists, capitulate to insurance company bureaucrats, or avoid the company that stands behind the AI algorithm.

Both pharmacists and prescribing physicians are advised to use computer-generated red flags only as calls-to-action to further review details in the patient's prescription history in conjunction with other relevant patient health information. They are told that red flags are not meant to supplant clinical judgment. But going against AI-generated results puts many providers at legal risk should an untoward event occur, and many may not want to accept that risk.

The entire scenario is somewhat Kafkaesque. It reminds me of The Who's anthemic song "Won't Get Fooled Again," which contains the classic line: "Meet the new boss, same as the old boss." Given the over-reliance on algorithmic-based AI, will the future of medicine give way to a new boss who is worse than the old boss? Let's not be fooled into thinking it can't happen. Simply read JL Lycette's *The Algorithm Will See You Now*, a near-future medical thriller that convincingly demonstrates the potential dangers of AI when technology is used beyond the boundaries of ethical practice. We should realize that AI-driven algorithms can only provide recommendations and cannot replace the judgment of clinicians who should be the ultimate decision makers.

To be sure, AI has produced some great achievements. But when patients are at the mercy of uncaring, unethical, and unsympathetic medical decision makers, aided by predictive algorithms built on proxy measures for public health that may or may not be associated with known clinical risk factors nor vetted by the FDA or other regulatory authorities, many patients will continue to suffer needlessly with increased pain and decreased quality of life.

Human Touch and Scientific Veracity Are Missing in Healthcare Technology

*Technology-based enhancements in triage and treatment
are coming dangerously close to replacing the wisdom
and guidance of experienced healthcare professionals.
Healthcare organizations need to recognize that "tools"
may compliment patient care, but they are not a
substitute for human interaction, judgment, and empathy.*

PHYSICIANS WHO WORKED REMOTELY during the coronavirus
pandemic were immersed in technology, perhaps accelerating its
integration with medical practice, but not necessarily its acceptance
or authenticity.

I tend to doubt the veracity of much of what I read in electronic
health care records. I also question reports based on data gleaned
from large medical databases, such as summaries about physician
compensation and practice trends.

Many reports that profile physicians are generated on professional websites independently or with the aid of self-anointed
"high-tech" companies. They verge on self-promotion, and the
integrity of the data may be compromised and deemed too unreliable
to be credible.

The adage "you can't always believe what you read" is truer today
than it ever was, and studies have shown that a great deal of medical
information on the internet is incorrect or misinforms the public.

Data collected to evaluate practice patterns may be incomplete.
The sampling methodology may be biased. "White papers" rarely
undergo peer review and often lack statistical review and analysis.
Observations frequently substitute for ironclad facts.

For example, Doximity published a report (April 9, 2023) comparing the top specialties chosen by students at my medical school alma mater in 1980 — my year of graduation — with the top specialties chosen by students in the 2023 graduating class. I noticed a few inconsistencies, so I sounded the alarm to the website's "support specialist."

The specialist replied, "Thank you so much for your suggestions and feedback about this data report. We have passed your message to our product team for review. We're always working to make our tools as useful as possible for physicians."

In a Machiavellian moment, I recalled Henry David Thoreau's prophetic statement in *Walden*: "Men have become the tools of their tools." Let's not let it happen, I said to myself.

Then I realized Thoreau's words have already rung true, considering the alarming number of problems associated with electronic health records: increased provider time, computer downtime, interrupted interactions with patients, lack of standards, and threats to confidentiality.

The reliability of the medical record has plummeted due to errors in documentation caused in part by input from multiple users and "copy and paste" errors.

In my specialty of psychiatry, virtual mental health startups are commonplace (essay 56). Most are privately funded. The companies seem to be infatuated with technology and boast of their ability to "democratize" mental health services by reaching millions of patients.

However, digital mental health care companies feel sterile and can be counterproductive to the benefits of in-person psychiatric treatment.

Mental health companies that function 100% online may be necessary to access patients in remote locations or when demand is high, but the distance exposes patients — now referred to as "clients" — to the ever-increasing dangers of virtual psychiatric treatment: unanswered pleas for help — occasionally from suicidal patients — and inappropriate prescribing of controlled substances.

Working at investor-backed telehealth startups has been chaotic and confusing and compared to working at fast-food chains. A whistleblower alleges that policies and practices at one company may have put profits and growth before patient safety.

It's telling that companies that provide virtual psychiatric services embed legal disclaimers in their websites explaining that services performed are only administrative, financial, and supportive. The fine print also makes it clear that their services do not address emergencies, and their providers are an addition to, and not a replacement for, local primary care providers.

The new breed of tele-mental health companies cites positive outcomes in patients who use their services. Patient testimonials adorn their websites, and once again debatable — surely, not statistically significant measurements — are designated as de facto indicators of clinical improvement.

I'm a stickler for medical protocol and accuracy because, after working a dozen years in the pharmaceutical industry, I saw how advertising statements could be easily manipulated and twisted for business purposes and wind up becoming false claims.

Claims made by online healthcare companies — on television, social media, and on their websites — should receive the same scientific scrutiny as pharmaceutical claims when they come before the FDA. All claims of efficacy must be truthful and not misleading, supported by robust statistical analyses.

I am not a Luddite. I've seen first-hand the benefits of technology when used constructively in pharma. The collective shift toward decentralization — conducting a portion or all of the clinical trial at patients' homes — coupled with investment in technological innovations that make home visits and data collection possible is changing the face of clinical trial development.

However, I am against using unproven or inferior technology with glitches that jeopardize patients' welfare. There is not, and probably will never be, an all-in-one, digital-only technology enterprise that allows providers to enter findings and diagnoses, take advantage of links that connect these with decision support modules and the medical literature, and communicate with colleagues and others taking care of the patient without some semblance of human touch and the eventual need for real-time intervention. Treatment cannot be provided indefinitely in cyberspace.

Clinician involvement is crucial for successfully designing and implementing medical applications and electronic health records. Clinicians must likewise step up and be visible in digital environments. Care received solely through online messaging is perilously being promoted as just as good as that provided in the office despite the huge differences between the two modalities and a bevy of limitations associated with mental health teletherapy.

Non-clinician-based digital mental health services like chatbots, video and written content, gamified user exercises, and digital cognitive behavioral therapy programs will never substitute for clinician-based, face-to-face treatment. No matter how much a physician's job can be replaced or aided by technology, the human touch will always remain a prerequisite for patient care.

There's More to Medical Practice than Meets the Eye

Physicians who conduct utilization review, serve as expert witnesses, or collaborate with advanced practice providers give medical advice and assert medical opinions. Their activities could be construed as the practice of medicine and therefore subject to disciplinary and/or malpractice proceedings in the event the information provided is egregious or harmful to patients.

Essay 48 addresses the imprecise and outdated nature of the definition of "medical practice." Court cases have continually changed the meaning and scope of practice. The following is an example of a typically vague and outdated state statute defining the term: "'Practice of medicine' or 'medical practice' means all activities authorized by a physician's and surgeon's certificate...."

Other definitions of medical practice, or what constitutes a medical practice, have been equally archaic. Physicians in Rhode Island concluded: "We need more information about medical practices in the state — much more information — and we need to begin by defining what we mean by 'a medical practice.' In fact, we may need more than one definition, as the answer to the question 'what is a medical practice?' varies according to why the question is asked, and for what the answer will be used."

The ambiguity in defining medical practice has led to a broadening of its interpretation over time and has opened new avenues of litigation against physicians who believed they were rendering administrative services, while courts instead found them involved in the treatment of patients, if only peripherally. Three areas of "medical practice" have recently come under scrutiny:

Utilization Review (UR): UR physicians render opinions about whether actual or proposed treatment and services are medically necessary. They work for insurance companies and third-party administrators, and they rarely have direct contact with patients, conferring instead with treating physicians. Nevertheless, their decisions are highly influential and often obstruct treatment or cause harm to patients.

The AMA's Prior Authorization and Utilization Management Reform Principles are 21 standards that address clinical validity, continuity of care, transparency and fairness, timely access and administrative efficiency, and alternatives and exemptions to UR. However, the document is silent about the role of UR physicians and the context in which UR decisions are made.

One must turn to individually litigated cases to determine whether UR activities constitute the practice of medicine. These cases are usually brought before the court by plaintiffs (patients or their families) injured by UR denials. The outcomes of such cases do not provide a consensus or consistent pattern of reasoning among the courts as to whether UR calibrates with medical practice.

Increasingly, however, physicians are put on the hot spot for their UR decisions, not only by plaintiff's attorneys, but also by state medical boards responsible for regulating the practice of medicine. Medical boards tend to view UR as an activity under their purview. Physicians should beware recruiters who attempt to lure them into UR jobs by advertising that UR companies are involved strictly in medical review and do not practice medicine because they do not provide medical care or form doctor-patient relationships. The argument just does not hold water.

Expert Witness: Similar to UR physicians, doctors who submit expert opinions in writing or provide expert witness testimony at depositions or in court may influence medical outcomes in the absence of a formal doctor-patient relationship. Although expert witnesses are typically utilized in malpractice cases, some testify in areas indirectly related to patient care — for example, physician peer review, worker's compensation, and product liability.

According to the AMA, whenever physicians serve as expert witnesses, they must accurately represent their qualifications, testify honestly, avoid personal and financial conflicts of interest, ensure their testimony is evidence-based, and testify only in areas in which they have been trained. Physicians should also have recent, substantive clinical experience and knowledge and not be "hired guns." The operative word is "recent."

The most effective (and credible) expert witnesses still see patients, at least part-time, and thus there is little debate whether providing testimony is an extension of their practice. Medical licensing boards may discipline physicians for providing false or misleading testimony or claims that are patently false.

Collaborating Physician: Entering into collaborative agreements with advanced practice providers (APPs), such as nurse practitioners and physician assistants, has become common as APPs have proliferated over the past two decades. APPs are often required to have formal agreements with supervising physicians. The failure of physicians to properly supervise APPs may be viewed as a breach of duty and serve as the basis for a negligence lawsuit in the event a patient suffers an adverse incident during treatment with an APP.

Physician supervision is more than a paperwork requirement. The duties of collaborating physicians are separate yet integral to medical practice insofar as collaborating physicians are consultants to APPs. Written agreements stipulate that collaborating physicians may be responsible for evaluating the performance of APPs, reviewing their medical records, cosigning their charts, and providing clinical oversight. Florida law clearly states that supervising physicians are responsible and liable for the performance and the acts and omissions of APPs.

Defining the practice of medicine can be elusive. The field is dynamic and continues to evolve. The evidence suggests that conducting utilization review, providing expert witness testimony, and collaborating with APPs falls within the realm of practicing medicine. All activities are subject to regulation by state licensing boards and are fodder for the legal system.

Because the scope of medical practice is viewed through a wide lens, many jobs previously considered non-clinical or non-traditional now require medical licenses. The North Carolina Medical Board warned that "patient harm can occur when physicians practicing outside areas in which they were trained are unable to meet accepted and prevailing standards of care in the new practice area."

It seems incredulous that a 1901 editorial in *JAMA* foreshadowed today's expanded interpretations of medical practice. A bill was before the New York legislature to amend the medical practice law by adding: "Any person shall be regarded as practicing medicine... who shall prescribe, direct, recommend, or advise, for the use of any person, any remedy or agent...for the treatment, relief or cure of any wound, fracture or bodily injury, infirmity, physical or mental, or other defect or disease."

The operative word is "advise" — and perhaps "recommend" and "direct" as well.

ESSAY 70

Gil-Scott Heron's "Winter in America" Is Upon Us

Moral injury, burnout, and depletion are characteristic of work in health systems today. If your motivation is a desire to care for patients, it may seem that your aspirations have become frozen. Who'll pay reparations for the great damage to our profession caused by the medical-industrial complex?

FOR ME, THE CHEERFUL MUSICAL SOUNDS of the holiday season invariably give way to a somber song: Gil Scott-Heron's "Winter in America." Dubbed the "Godfather of Rap," Gil Scott-Heron (1949–2011) embraced diverse musical styles alternating between jazz, blues, soul, and hip-hop. He wasn't known for delivering good tidings as much as he was for sermonizing and engaging in "Small Talk at 125th and Lenox," inquiring, "Who'll Pay Reparations on My Soul?"

"Winter in America" appeared on Scott-Heron's 1975 album The First Minute of a New Day, a collaboration with his college classmate Brian Jackson, who was also musical arranger, pianist, and flautist. "Winter in America" the song is often confused with "Winter in America" the record album released by Scott-Heron and Jackson a year earlier; however, the song had not yet been written, so it is not found on the album that bears its name. Both the song and the album deal with socially conscious, racially tinged themes affecting the plight of marginalized African Americans and urban dwellers in the late 1960s and early to mid-1970s.

Scott-Heron would often introduce the song "Winter in America" in concert by saying that winter "got mad" and decided to stay, pushing aside the other seasons, not in terms of the climate but rather the philosophy, politics, and psychology of the day. Scott-Heron believed America was at a standstill, a time when "all the healers have been killed or been betrayed." It was a time when no one was fighting for socio-political causes because "nobody knows what to save." "Winter in America" became a metaphor for frozen dreams, promises, and aspirations — dashed hopes of meaningful societal change to overcome racism and other forms of oppression.

Fast-forward almost 50 years and we have yet to realize brighter times and warmer days. Physicians have become enslaved by systems of all kinds, ranging from electronic to corporate. Approximately 20% of physicians will leave medicine by the end of 2023. Most practitioners acknowledge suffering some form of moral injury during the pandemic, trying to do their best but stymied by those in power, much like the healers in "Winter in America" who felt betrayed or "were sent away."

To be clear, "Winter in America" was not written with the medical profession in mind. However, the politically charged nature of the song speaks to themes of governance apropos medical practice. As I have maintained elsewhere, politics and politicians have come to dominate medical agendas, controlling what passes for scientific fact and "evidence."

"Winter in America" foreshadowed the politicization of medicine described in essays 49 and 50. Scott-Heron noted that the Constitution is merely a "noble piece of paper." Cannot the same be said about practice guidelines discarded due to science denialism? Black poets like Gil Scott-Heron were the news-givers of his era because they believed their stories were not covered truthfully by the mainstream media.

Political corruption was a favorite topic of Scott-Heron. In "The Revolution Will Not Be Televised," arguably Scott-Heron's most famous song, he raps: "You will not be able to stay home, brother. You will not be able to plug in, turn on and cop out. You will not be able to lose yourself on skag and skip out for beer during commercials because the revolution will not be televised." A revolution, like medical practice, must be experienced.

Scott-Heron's "H2Ogate Blues" targeted "King Richard" Nixon (among other autocrats). The song asks, "Just how blind will America be" to trickery and dishonesty in politics? Do we not sometimes wonder the same thing about individuals in charge of health care policy, given the widening gap in health inequity in the United States today?

"'B' Movie" and "Re-Ron" heavily criticized Ronald Reagan's economic initiatives and his 1984 re-election campaign. Healthcare was negatively impacted by Reaganomics. As noted by music analyst Ben Sisario, "With sharp, sardonic wit and a barrage of pop-culture references, [Gil Scott-Heron] derided society's dominating forces as well as the gullibly dominated." However, the elderly, disabled, young children, and the poor all suffered under the Reagan administration's cost-cutting policies. They were helpless victims too innocent to be considered "gullible."

Scott-Heron's biting commentaries were delivered through a broad lens of poetry, novels, and song lyrics. Many were relevant to medical practice. Topics included social injustice ("Whitey on the Moon"), civil rights ("Johannesburg"), substance use ("Angel Dust"), and nuclear technology ("We Almost Lost Detroit"). Some of Scott-Heron's most memorable performances occurred in 1979 in a series of anti-nuclear themed concerts in New York City organized by the likes of Jackson Browne, Bonnie Raitt, and John Hall under the auspices of Musicians United for Safe Energy, a.k.a. the MUSE "No Nukes" benefit concerts.

While doctors were not directly the subjects of Scott-Heron's songs, they figured prominently in a few, most notably "The Bottle." The song is told via a series of vignettes connected only by alcohol. A young boy running scared from his drunken father; a woman turning to alcohol and violence after her boyfriend is imprisoned; and (seemingly) an abortion doctor drinking away his shame.

Although Scott-Heron was keen to point out the harm of addictive substances, he was unable to resist the urges himself. In "Home is Where the Hatred Is," Scott-Heron delivers a sobering reality check to anyone who has struggled with addiction and to their healers: "You keep saying, kick it, quit it, kick it, quit it. God, did you ever try to turn your sick soul inside out so that the world could watch you die?"

Scott-Heron did try to quit drugs (mainly crack cocaine), but unfortunately, substance use overcame him and his career imploded. Whereas he recorded over a dozen albums between 1970 and 1982, Scott-Heron released only two albums thereafter. He rarely performed in his later years, partly because he was incarcerated and because his teeth were missing and decayed (likely due to cocaine) which affected his pronunciation.

The exact cause of Scott-Heron's death in 2011 was never revealed, but he disclosed in a 2008 interview with New York magazine that he had been living with HIV for several years. In "I'm New Here," his final recording made a year prior to his death, Scott-Heron penned, "New York is Killing Me," hinting at physicians who underestimated his condition: "Bunch of doctors coming round, they don't know that New York is killing me."

Scott-Heron was honored posthumously with a Grammy Lifetime Achievement Award in 2012, and in 2021 he was inducted into the Rock and Roll Hall of Fame as a recipient of the Early Influence Award.

"Winter in America" — the song and the album — is considered one of the greatest political statements on record, literally and figuratively. According to the British journalist and author Dylan Jones, "Scott-Heron was Curtis Mayfield, Malcolm X, and James Brown rolled into one: radical campaigner, accomplished musician, professional nuisance, compelling poet." No doubt he would have made a formidable physician as well.

Are Physicians with MBAs Traitors to Healthcare?

Most physicians with MBA degrees perceive their business education as a valuable investment they would pursue again even with the high financial and opportunity cost of an MBA. Contrary to concerns that dual-degree physicians are disinterested in clinical care, the vast majority leverage their new perspectives and skills to improve healthcare delivery.

LET ME BE COMPLETELY UPFRONT. I have an MD degree and an MBA degree. I earned my medical degree in 1980 and my business degree in 1996. I wrote the first definitive textbook about physicians with dual degrees (MD/MBA). Subsequently, I've written many papers on the topic, and I maintain articles and news clippings in several file folders each 3 to 4 inches thick. I keep track of current trends. I encourage medical students and early career physicians to apply to business school if they have a genuine interest in the business and management aspects of medical practice.

However, the topic of dual-degree physicians easily unnerves me. I am sensitive to unkind remarks made about physicians with MD (or DO) and MBA degrees. I wrote an op-ed about "faking" my way through medical school (essay 35) and a physician responded, "I believe that the author who has by his name, MD and MBA, suggests he likely never was made for medicine." What a sanctimonious doctor!

Physicians have been seeking MBA degrees for decades. Both the number of executive MBA programs and the number of MD/ MBA programs offered by medical schools has steadily increased, as has the number of physicians receiving MBA degrees from these programs. The trend first became newsworthy in 1994, when *The Wall Street Journal* published an article with the title "A New Breed of M.D.s Add M.B.A. to Vitae," written by George Anders.

Anders appeared to have penned the piece believing that, based on his interview sources, adding an MBA degree to one's MD degree was a way to enhance physicians' marketability and allow them to "pivot quickly ... between the world of stethoscopes and the world of spreadsheets." An MBA degree was viewed as a "ticket to open doors" and put doctors on a fast-track for hospital leadership positions. Physicians' motivation for obtaining MBA degrees today remains basically the same as it did 30 years ago: to learn more about the business of healthcare and prepare them for taking on additional administrative responsibilities.

Several years after *The Wall Street Journal* article was published, the late distinguished physician Leonard Laster, MD, wrote the book *Life After Medical School*. In the book, Laster categorized and described five basic career pathways in medicine: primary care, surgery, psychiatry, disciplines removed from ongoing patient care (anesthesiology, pathology, radiology and nuclear medicine), and areas that bear little if any relationship to medical practice, such as management and politics.

Further thoughts about the fifth career pathway — pursuits distanced from clinical medicine — led Laster to write a scathing article in 1998 in the now defunct *American Medical News*, which served as the official publication of the American Medical Association. The article was titled "Physicians with MBAs? Not my doctor!" Laster opined that physicians cannot — and should not — serve two masters, concluding, "I will not allow my family members to be guinea pigs for testing whether these professional polarities [medicine and business] can be successfully used. I say let businessmen be businessmen and pursue profits, and let doctors be doctors and care for patients."

Laster's op-ed enraged readers and generated more letters to the editor than any article previously published in *American Medical News*. Obstetrician/gynecologist G.V. Raghu, MD, wrote a letter expressing the sentiments of many physicians who responded to

Laster's commentary. Raghu wrote, "It is amazing that Leonard Laster, MD...looks at MBA training as an antithesis of medical values. Does he prefer nonphysician MBAs to be making the management, cost-cutting and quality management decisions?" Dr. Raghu — and many physicians since 1998 — have thoughtfully made the case that dual-degree physicians would be a positive influence on how care is delivered.

The great debate about physicians with MBAs thus became entrenched in articles and letters, with definitive data lacking to answer the question whether an MBA degree adds real value for physicians or forces them to live by two incompatible creeds. In the continued absence of such data and notwithstanding the perceived value of an MBA degree including larger salaries for dual-degree physicians, the debate still rages.

Many academicians consider dual-degree physicians traitors to the medical profession despite research showing that business skills do not, in fact, lower practice competencies or draw students away from medicine. I've had to counsel several entrepreneurial medical school applicants and advise them to curb their enthusiasm about business school lest the interviewer reject them outright. I'm not convinced there is ever a good time for medical students and residents to declare their interest in business school. For various reasons, they may benefit by waiting until after residency to pursue an MBA degree.

Fortunately, a few level-headed and well-respected academicians have chimed in to even the debate. One, in particular, is my good friend and colleague David Nash, MD, MBA, founder and dean emeritus of the Jefferson College of Population Health in Philadelphia, Pennsylvania. In 1986, Nash and two colleagues anticipated the need for management-trained physicians to lead the "medical industrial complex." In their article published in *The New England Journal of Medicine*, they did not specify the importance of a business degree, but they argued that physicians needed additional training in management theory, educated perhaps through professional organizations.

In 1999, Thomas Bodenheimer, MD and Lawrence Casalino, MD, PhD wrote a two-part article for *The New England Journal of Medicine* apparently legitimizing the role of "[physician] executives with white coats." They described various roles and responsibilities of HMO medical directors. But in doing so, they continued the debate started by Laster.

Bodenheimer and Casalino wrote: "The two opposing views reflect inherent conflicts in the role of medical directors – between the desires of patients and physicians, on the one hand, and the financial profit or survival of the organization, on the other, and between the unlimited demands of individual patients and the limited resources of society." Simply put, business-minded physicians are — and always will be — stuck between medicine and management.

Diana Chapman Walsh, president emeritus of Wellesley College, published her PhD thesis as a book about corporate physicians. She offers a management lesson not taught in medical or business school — one that needs to be learned through experience and deep personal reflection: Physicians must learn how to manage the tension that exists between their obligations as doctors and their role as part of management.

This applies equally to physicians working for organizations and those who are self-employed. Unless this underlying conflict is appropriately handled, as I discuss in the next essay, physicians risk harm to their patients and reputations, and they may remain unpopular with their colleagues.

When an MBA Degree Meets Medicine: An Eye-Opening Experience

Consider this essay a continuation of the previous one,
highlighting conflicts between medicine and business.
Given the unusual path of physicians with MBA degrees,
people aren't always clear about their intentions.

In early 2023, I saw an ophthalmologist for my worsening eyesight. The doctor came highly recommended and was credentialed as an MD and MBA. He founded his practice, which has grown to over a dozen practitioners. His website boasts how he works with the pharmaceutical industry to help develop and market new medications "that improve the standard of care."

According to Open Payments data, the doctor has relationships with 10 drug companies and received nearly $20,000 total compensation in 2021 — 60% for consulting fees and the remainder for honoraria, travel, lodging, food, and beverage. His industry payments since 2015 have been well above the U.S. mean and the mean for his specialty.

I googled the physician before my appointment. The feedback was generally positive, with occasional references to patients feeling rushed or being pushed into surgery. My exam lasted approximately three minutes. The doctor told me I had "dry eyes" and gave me sample medications marketed by companies with whom he had relationships. Then came the bombshell: The doctor told me I needed cataract surgery. I decided to seek a second opinion. It pains me to admit it, but I wished the doctor did not have an MBA degree or industry ties.

My pain stems from the fact that I'm guilty on both accounts. Not only do I have an MBA degree, I also worked in the pharmaceutical industry. While working in big pharma, I gave many promotional talks to physicians and visited "key opinion leaders" — that is, physicians of influence — keeping them abreast of products in the pipeline and current scientific research so they could pass the knowledge on to other physicians.

Should I apologize for my activities? Should I think less of the ophthalmologist? I don't think so. Both of us have conflicts. Conflicts are universal in medicine. It's not the declaration of conflicts that's important, it's how you manage them. Rule number one for managing conflicts of interest is to be aware of them. They're like the blind spots I discussed in essay 4: Our conflicts diminish as we develop greater insight about ourselves and begin to behave ethically. Personal integrity cannot be taught in medical or business school.

It's often assumed that doctors with MBAs have sold out to big business or are at least mired in conflict. I'm not convinced that's true. The fact is, I sought a second ophthalmological opinion for my own peace of mind, to ensure the initial recommendation for surgery was based on the ophthalmologist's obligation to me as his patient and not on his role as a practice owner or pharmaceutical consultant or thought leader.

The reality is that an MBA degree creates value and opens doors to new opportunities. More than ever, job descriptions will state an MBA degree is a "plus." There is no doubt that healthcare organizations are in search of business-minded physicians capable of leading the "medical industrial complex." A salary premium comes with a dual degree. Perhaps most important, MBA-trained physicians understand the language of business, just as medical students are taught the language of medicine. Fears that an MBA degree will draw physicians away from practice are unfounded.

Soon after I obtained my MBA, I wrote a book about dual-degree physicians: MDs and DOs with MBA degrees. A good friend and colleague, Kenneth Veit, DO, MBA, was an "early adaptor" and turned me on to the idea of business school. I asked him to contribute a chapter to the book, specifically addressing the value of an MBA degree to someone in his position: Dean of the Philadelphia College of Osteopathic Medicine (now emeritus).

Veit said his decision to go to business school came about with a slowly developing interest in administration. He wrote: "[An] MBA education can be applied to [operational] interactions.... The MBA skills constantly function in the background. When the occasion calls, this database of knowledge moves to the foreground ... [An MBA degree] provides a set of skills that is rarely directly applicable but that at the same time is constantly being used indirectly in various formats."

A 2021 published survey of 66 dual-degree orthopedic surgeons provided additional insight. They were asked about their motivations for obtaining an MBA degree and its perceived value. Most respondents (89.4%) viewed the MBA degree as either extremely valuable or valuable. Their time spent in administrative activities significantly increased — consistent with their goals — and business school allowed them to focus on learning important management theory considered a prerequisite for leading health care systems undergoing change.

I utilized my MBA degree in a somewhat different capacity while working in the pharmaceutical industry. I had an opportunity to dive deeply into marketing while in business school, and I decided to put that knowledge to good use in big pharma. I trained sales teams and reviewed all types of promotional material — for physicians and consumers — for medical accuracy, completeness, and realism.

Working as an "insider," I guarded against potential FDA violations and was able to boost the credibility of advertising claims in areas where pharmaceutical companies struggle mightily: incurring fines for false or misleading prescription drug promotion. I was asked, "Why do you stoop to popularizing medicine?" The answer rolled off my tongue: "Because advances made in the lab cannot benefit people without actions taken outside the lab."

Butting heads with the "suits," however, was another matter. I understood profit and loss as well as they did. I was adept at reading financial statements. I understood forecasting models; heck, I formulated models in business school. One of my professors told the class he loves to make models for fun. We thought he was talking about replica cars!

Pharma politics eventually wore me down. But that's not why I left my first job in pharma. I was asked by a salesperson to speak at a "lunch 'n learn" at an academic medical center to promote a new drug for depression. I met the salesperson in the parking lot. He had a half-dozen large pizza boxes to bring to the conference room. I offered to carry some boxes. We entered the room together. The faculty mistook me for the salesperson.

The lyrics to Chris Trapper's song "Keg On My Coffin" were forever seared into my memory:

> "Drink up life like a river
> 'til the pizza man delivers
> And smile and know
> I loved you 'til the end."

It wasn't the "end" of me, but I realized that being mistaken for a pizza man signaled I was too deep in the big pharma marketing machinery (see essay 42), so I left the company for a more respectable position in R&D. Still, I lent my skills to marketing teams throughout my pharmaceutical career, including generating ideas for television commercials. My MBA degree put me on a level playing field. And who other than a psychiatrist was more qualified to advise a director and actor how to portray a patient with schizophrenia or bipolar disorder?

Medicine Is a Joke, Except No One Is Laughing

A tale of a near-apocalyptical ending
to the medical profession.

MY BROTHER AND I LIKE TO SWAP STORIES about our medical experiences. I suppose our ages — 69 for me and 74 for him — lead to varied encounters and tales.

"It's a sh*t-show," he tells me on the phone from his home on Martha's Vineyard. "No one's left here on the island. The doctors who remain have stopped seeing new patients or have incredibly long waiting lists." My brother is forced to go to medical centers in Boston to see doctors.

It's not the shortage of physicians that irks him, however. It's the impersonal way healthcare is delivered plus the fact that telemedicine isn't the panacea it's cracked up to be, certainly not when physical and neurological exams are required to evaluate his fused lumbar spine and painful and progressive neuropathy.

"Now it's my turn to complain," I tell him. I describe how providing care to patients is a sacred trust built on meaningful relationships. However, that trust, and the rapport between doctors and patients, is being eroded by the technological accoutrements of contemporary practice.

I relate how artificial intelligence is revamping the future of medical practice, from the chatbot known as ChatGPT (essay 67) to apps that can easily be installed on computers and smart mobile devices. For example, when I logged in to my medical chart through a patient portal to send my PCP a message, a pop-up screen appeared before the message could be delivered:

- Call 911 if you have an emergency.
- Allow up to two business days for a medical question response.

- For new problems, including skin conditions, use Symptom Checker or schedule an appointment before sending a message (both "Symptom Checker" and "schedule and appointment" were hyperlinked).
- Messages to your provider are part of your medical record.

I was curious to learn about Symptom Checker, so I clicked on the hyperlink, which first directed me to the "Terms and Use." I pretended to understand legalese and then I was introduced to Symptom Checker.

Here is what the bot offered:

"Welcome to Symptom Checker! Tell us how you're feeling, and we'll help you get the right care, including:

eVisit

If your symptoms are minor, you might be able to complete an eVisit right away. You'll just have to answer a few questions about your symptoms, and a health care provider will send a diagnosis and treatment plan to your inbox.

Urgent care video visit

Some minor conditions don't require in-person care, but do require a face-to-face conversation with a provider. In those cases, we'll help you start a video visit and get the care you need from the comfort of home.

Urgent care or doctor's office

If your condition is minor but requires in-person care, we'll help you find an urgent care near you or schedule a visit with your doctor.

Emergency room

If your symptoms are life-threatening, call 911 or seek emergency care right away."

A few things strike me as both funny and tragic about the messages. First, the healthcare system doesn't want me to see my PCP. It prefers instead to shield him with a chatbot acting like a downfield line blocker.

Second, the health system puts the onus squarely on me, aided by minimal advice, to figure out if my condition requires an in-person visit. The proverbial cart is before the horse insofar as triage is suggested before a diagnosis is made.

Third, a dummy understands to call 911 if they are experiencing a life-threatening emergency. I am not a dummy.

Lastly, all I needed from my PCP was a refill of medication.

Nevertheless, I clicked on the Symptom Checker to explore the application. I was asked to pick the symptom or condition that most closely matched what I had been experiencing. The artificially unintelligent program generated over two-dozen conditions to self-treat or self-medicate with OTC drugs. The conditions ranged from sunburn to rash to athlete's foot to jock itch to constipation and even COVID-19. Once again, the goal was to spare the health system an unnecessary PCP visit.

I clicked on "Mental Health," because at this point, I thought I might need to see a psychiatrist. I was advised to call the Suicide & Crisis Lifeline (988) if I am in crisis.

Next, I was asked to enter my phone number and questioned whether I was thinking about hurting myself or someone else. Responding in the negative, I was asked if I am either (1) sad; (2) anxious or worried; or (3) unusually happy, excited, or hyper. Choosing none of these options, I was offered an urgent video call. However, endorsing manic-like symptoms (happy, excited, hyper) simply suggested that I make an appointment with my PCP.

Now I felt like hurting someone. The algorithm was clinically flawed. It didn't recognize hypomania or mania as a psychiatric emergency. Furthermore, when I endorsed "sad" or "anxious and worried," I was required to take the PHQ-9 and GAD-7 screening instruments for depression and anxiety, respectively. These screens, although commonly used in mental health and primary care settings, are far from perfect. Interpreting their results at face value without the benefit of a clinical evaluation can have detrimental consequences for patients in terms of false positives and negatives.

I played along and endorsed severe depressive symptoms on the PHQ-9. I was advised to contact my PCP. Ironically, Dr. Symptom Checker further burdens PCPs by designating them to be on point for patients' mental health problems. This is especially egregious considering that my PCP practices in a health system that has a psychiatry department. Why aren't their mental health services integrated with primary care, as is best practice?

The over-reliance on and uncertainty of artificial intelligence is one of myriad problems plaguing health delivery systems. Add to those problems the depersonalization and dehumanization of the medical experience and you have a recipe for ... well, as my brother put it: "a sh*t-show." And let's not forget about the increasingly intolerable conditions under which physicians must practice: toxic workplaces, EHR calamities, and nonstop hounding by third parties (essay 51), to name a few.

Medical practice has become a joke, staffed by threadbare providers, possibly not even human. Physicians who remain loyal to the cause are not laughing, however. They are burning out at record rates — 40% higher than workers in other fields — and dealing with moral injury inflicted by deceptive health systems that dangle lucrative employment contracts promising to honor physicians' beliefs and values, only to find they were sold a false bill of goods. What was once a sacred pledge taken by physicians to uphold the sanctity and standards of the medical profession now rests uncomfortably on the shoulders of healthcare managers and software engineers with limited knowledge and understanding of clinical practice.

Although physicians clearly feel a moral imperative to spend time forming important human connections, inherent transactional demands of health systems have undermined these ideals. A strong bond between doctors and their patients, once considered a *sine qua non* for healing, no longer endures. All that remains are reflections from a golden era of medicine before technology displaced grace and, along with it, the dignity and pride of physicians who were summoned to heal.

How Can There Be Joy in Medicine if There Is No Joy in Mudville?

In The Field of Dreams, Terence Mann (James Earl Jones)
remarks, "The one constant through all the years ... has
been baseball." What of the future of medicine?

THE CLASSIC POEM "CASEY AT THE BAT" delves into the dashed dreams of 5,000 frenzied fans who gathered to watch the "Mudville nine" play baseball, pinning their hopes on their star player, Casey. Do they have unrealistic expectations of Casey, or is his prowess over-hyped? And what implications does this time-honored poem have for medical practice?

Parables — short stories that teach a moral or spiritual lesson — are powerful tools in medicine (see essay 58). "Casey at the Bat" is no exception. Although it is often considered a poem, "Casey" is actually a ballad (stories in rhyme), written by Ernest Lawrence Thayer, a columnist for *The San Francisco Examiner* newspaper. Thayer wrote the ballad in two hours and was paid five dollars for it. "Casey at the Bat: A Ballad of the Republic Sung in the Year 1888," as it was officially designated, was published on June 3, 1888. The poem became famous similar to the way new prescription drugs and results of medical studies reach the public: through dissemination by the media.

"Casey at the Bat" is set against a backdrop of "deep despair": fans who are desperate for Casey to get a whack at the ball, not unlike physicians who pray for miracles for their patients. Against all odds, with two outs in the final inning and two batters preceding him, Casey does, in fact, advance to home plate. The fans' prayers have been answered; the two players batting before Casey have amazingly reached base. The crowd — the "stricken multitude" — are rewarded and uplifted "to the wonderment of all."

Thayer writes: "There was ease in Casey's manner as he stepped into his place … No stranger in the crowd could doubt 'twas Casey at the bat." However, the team leader failed to deliver. Mighty Casey struck out. Casey's failure may have been due to one of several factors described by Robert M. Peters, MD, MBA, in his book *When Physicians Fail as Managers*, such as inadequate talent, poor training, lack of desire to get the job done and, most likely, impatience. Casey went down after only three pitches.

As a result of Casey's misadventure, there was no joy in Mudville. The sun stopped shining. The band stopped playing. Men stopped laughing. Children stopped shouting. Health disparities increased, especially among those who attended the game "from benches, black with people." Gloom and doom settled over the town so thick you could cut it with a knife.

Physicians who practiced in Mudville, many of them baseball fans, were deeply affected by the turn of events. In the game's wake, 43% reported they regretted choosing medicine as a career. They looked for scapegoats rather than blame Casey, and they cited the "suits," crying "fraud." The physicians discovered that the owners of the Mudville nine were penny-pinching businessmen who also owned the local hospital and many others in their for-profit chain. The owners' callous management was responsible for staffing shortages, incivility and high levels of moral distress, leading to burnout and depression among the majority of physicians who practiced in town.

With professional fulfillment at an all-time low, there was no way to make a difference and improve joy and meaning in their work. Psychiatrists who recalled Freud saying "love and work" were necessary ingredients for personal fulfillment were charged with breaking the bad news to their colleagues that one condition — work — was missing from their repertoire, and the other condition — love — was absent in a quarter, insofar as the divorce rate among physicians is approximately 25%.

Fortunately, the American Medical Association stepped up to the plate. Long considered an ineffectual organization unable to unionize the medical profession like professional sports, the AMA informed the physicians of Mudville that they had a "recovery plan," one intended to reduce physician burnout and provide resources that prioritize well-being and work conditions so physicians can focus on what really matters: patient care. The AMA even sponsored The Joy in Medicine™ Health System Recognition Program "designed to spark and guide organizations interested, committed or already engaged in improving physician satisfaction and reducing burnout."

Additional officialdoms such as The National Academy of Medicine and the Department of Health and Human Services, including the office of the U.S. Surgeon General, instituted measures to address burnout and cultivate professional fulfillment. You would think that all these resources would have restored joy to the physicians of Mudville. However, researchers found that professional fulfillment scores continued to fall. Perhaps we shouldn't blame Casey's ill-timed blow; maybe we just need more time to let all those esteemed organizations work their magic.

It's a little-known fact that "Casey at the Bat" was not immediately a fan-favorite. The poem gained additional notoriety when William DeWolf Hopper, a New York actor and sports fan, enacted the ballad during his stage routine. The crowd went wild, as they say in baseball vernacular, and soon newspapers and magazines across the country reprinted "Casey." It was only after Casey's tale was widely disseminated that the plight of the Mudville nine and its townspeople became famous. In fact, two cities in the U.S. laid claim to the name "Mudville" as their own.

If that doesn't bring a tear of joy to your eye, perhaps you *should* reconsider medicine as your calling.

Narrative Medicine Writing Saved My Sanity

*Mark Twain said don't let school interfere with
your education. But there are exceptions.*

STORYTELLING SAVED MY SANITY during the coronavirus pandemic.
The lockdown afforded me time to write the 74 essays that preceded
this one. I didn't imagine I was writing my memoir as much as I
was engaged in the practice of narrative medicine writing — telling
stories about the meaning of illness and reflecting on the vastness
and depth of human experience in the healthcare setting. Soon after I
began writing the essays, I discovered the field of narrative medicine
has been around since the turn of the century.

Rita Charon, MD, PhD is widely credited for originating the field
of narrative medicine. She inaugurated and teaches in the Master
of Science in Narrative Medicine graduate program at Columbia
University, where she received her PhD degree in English following her medical degree from Harvard. Charon is also co-author of
Principles and Practice of Narrative Medicine and other scholarly
works. In her seminal article on narrative medicine, published in *The
Journal of the American Medical Association* in 2001, Charon wrote:
"The effective practice of medicine requires narrative competence,
that is, the ability to acknowledge, absorb, interpret, and act on the
stories and plights of others."

Storytelling and writing competencies are taken for granted. But
the fact is that few narrative medicine writing programs actually
incorporate writing skills as a program goal, including medical
schools that have integrated medical humanities into their curricula,
which now number well over 100 in the U.S. The authors of the
most comprehensive review of narrative medicine writing programs
to date recommended expanding program objectives "to include the

development of enhanced writing skills and self-efficacy related to the writing process as measurable learning outcomes."

Laura Weiss Roberts, MD, MA, chair of psychiatry at Stanford University and editor-in-chief of *Academic Medicine,* and John Coverdale, MD, MEd, professor of psychiatry, behavioral sciences, and medical ethics at Baylor College of *Medicine*, observed that many gifted physicians "... struggle when it comes to writing. They fret. They delay. They feel inadequate – even inauthentic. While these colleagues may view teaching and healing as natural capacities, they view writing as anything but."

Perhaps some physicians need tools to write creatively — tools that can only be obtained through formal education. In my case, despite my penchant for writing, I realized I had virtually no formal education in writing and English literature. That's why I decided to enroll in a narrative medicine writing program at a local university. I'm taking several graduate-level courses leading to a "certificate" in narrative healthcare. Here is a list of the courses:

Introduction to Narrative Medicine: Narrative as a Form of Knowledge

"A study of readings by narratively trained practitioners as well as writing assignments that move practitioners beyond clinical knowledge into narrative knowledge. Through engagement with literature and writing, students develop comfort with the less-defined areas of care-the open spaces of provider-patient relationships where ethics, empathy, and the unknown hold more power than heart-rate and x-ray."

Narratives of Illness

"A study of illness narratives in poetry, short fiction, creative nonfiction, and novels. Emphasis on close reading and developing narrative competency and empathy."

Writing & Healing

"A study of narratives by doctors and other care providers. Emphasis on reflective writing skills as students develop their own narratives, addressing presence, complexity, paradox, fatigue, shame, love, listening, and other human facets of care."

One of the appealing features of this program is that classes can be taken in any order. Each class is three credit hours given for two hours one evening per week for 16 weeks (10 weeks during the summer). Courses are conducted remotely via Zoom. They are spaced out over three semesters and can be completed in about a year. Individuals choosing a more formal course of study leading to a Master of Fine Arts (MFA) in creative writing need to accumulate 36 additional credit hours (a total of 15 three-credit courses), which usually takes several years to complete.

At this stage of my life — turning 70 with an MBA degree in tow — I'm not keen on continuing my education beyond the basic nine-credit certificate program. However, one never knows. There are many enticing "supportive" workshops conducted at this university and courses designed to identify and apply rhetorical theory to various writing genres including poetry and fiction. At a cost of $690 per credit hour — or a minimum of $2,070 per course — I'll have to choose wisely should I decide to pursue my training beyond a certificate.

I was impressed by one physician, a cardiothoracic surgeon, who decided to take the plunge and shell out $31,050 for an MFA degree. The reason he gave for furthering his education was described in the university's marketing brochure. The surgeon commented, "Writing has helped me in more ways than I can count. I host a monthly Narrative Healthcare Seminar at our hospital which is very gratifying. I also think writing is an excellent way for physicians like me to prevent burnout and to focus on the deeper meaning of what we do and how we can enhance care for our patients." This physician has subsequently retired from practice and now holds himself as an author (six novels) and freelance writer on his LinkedIn profile — and he is in good company.

Jennifer Lycette, MD, is a hematology-oncology physician who doubles as a novelist and award-winning essayist (see essay 67). She gave an account on *KevinMD* (May 1, 2023) about how writing and storytelling helped her recover from burnout. By embracing her "writer's side," she was able to experience the one thing considered anathema to medical culture yet essential for her recovery: vulnerability. Lycette was able to return to practice precisely because writing helped her discover her "sensitive, authentic self," suppressed during training and practice.

Indeed, the benefits touted by narrative medicine programs, whether geared toward a certificate or master's degree, include enhancing narrative competence, communication and empathy; detecting and mitigating burnout; fostering reflection with regard to professional identity formation; promoting team building and facilitating teaching competencies. Interacting with highly engaged students in the health professions and energetic teachers — most of whom are accomplished authors and writers in their own right — creates an esprit de corps, a passion for a life of impact. The learning environment becomes a stimulus for the narrative.

My son is a writer and teaches creative writing to college students. When he was in graduate school, one of his professors remarked, "The best advice I can give you is to write every day whether you feel like it or not." The great science fiction writer Isaac Asimov was a compulsive writer. He said his idea of a good time was to go up to his attic and sit at his electric typewriter and bang away. Asimov reasoned, "If my doctor told me I only had 6 months to live, I wouldn't brood. I'd type a little faster."

AFTERWORD

On the Road to Discovery

"THE BALANCE TO FACT AND ANALYSIS IS FEELING," our narrative medicine writing instructor informs us. "You'll find that each poem and essay and story that you write reflects a new aspect of yourself. Be curious about what's going on. Allow new poems onto the page. Allow free writing in prose and poetry. You have worlds inside you."

And then, predictably, the homework assignment for next week: "Create and post your '800 words.' The word count is purely there to make writing into the void less intimidation. When we write, we open a portal to our inner life. Joseph Campbell calls it 'following the echoes of the eloquence within.' I love that. The challenge lies in trusting those echoes. It is related to trusting intuition. Allow. Allow. Allow. Trust. Trust. Trust. No matter how many classes I've taught, no matter how many poems I've written, no matter how many books I've read: every single new thing is just that. A new field to move into within myself. I never have any clue what I am doing."

Clueless. That's me, too. I'm not good at this stream of consciousness thing. But I should be. After all, I am a psychiatrist. I've been at this for more than 40 years – listening to my patients' free associations and reflecting on my own in therapy. And trust. What's that? Post-pandemic moral injury has all but obliterated trust.

Nevertheless, I am eager to learn more about this free-form process of creative writing and narrative medicine and how to follow my "echoes." So, I do what comes naturally to me: I research (Google) it. Except I'm told: *"No results found for Joseph Campbell 'following the echoes of the eloquence within.'"* But Google tells me that *Joseph Campbell* encourages the audience to discover what excites them, and to make that the basis for their personal journeys. That sounds exactly like what our instructor was trying to tell us.

I then stumble upon similar words of wisdom from Paul Simon. No one writes poems as creatively lyrical as Rhymin' Simon. "I'm more interested in what I discover than what I invent," Simon tells *American Songwriter*, discussing how he crafted "You Can Call Me Al." Asked what the distinction is between discovery and invention, he explains, "You just have *no* idea that that's a thought that you had; it surprises you; it can make me laugh or make me emotional. When it happens and I'm the audience and I react, I have faith in that because I'm already reacting. I don't have to question it. I've already been the audience. But if I make it up, knowing where it's going, it's not as much *fun*. It may be just as good, but it's more *fun* to discover it."

So that's the key to creative writing! Follow the yellow brick road, the one paved with dreams and aspirations, hopes and failures, love and kindness, betrayal and refuge, levity as well as gravitas. It's a long and winding road to be sure, maybe one with no terminus, or maybe one that, as our instructor imagines, "lies beyond, within and woven through the anatomy and physiology of life," adding: "In the words of Dr. Chris Adrian of the Columbia University Narrative Medicine Program, 'Narrative Medicine begins where medicine ends.'"

Now I am *really* curious. I follow this thread further in my research. I become immersed in discovery much like Paul Simon. Hell. I *am* Paul Simon. I am on a father and son journey to Graceland. Simon tells *American Songwriter*: "The song [Graceland] started to write itself. It became a narrative … and Graceland became more like a metaphor than an actual destination."

I begin to travel along this metaphorical path. It is a path familiar to purists in the field of literary medicine, those who distinguish between "narrative medicine" and "narrative practice." Following Simon, I, too, begin to see "angels in the architecture." They're "spinning in infinity." Hallelujah!

There's one stop remaining on my journey, however. I am at the doorstep of Cat "Yusuf" Stevens, who, like Simon, has set out on a voyage of self-discovery, to clear his mind and see what he can discover "On the Road to Find Out." Stevens was not writing about traveling in a literal sense but instead bent on finding out who he was and the purpose, if any, of his existence. The last couplet of the song is revelatory:

The answer lies within, so why not take a look now?
Kick out the Devil's sin, pick up, pick up a good book now.

A dozen books have been assigned to us. Narrative medicine and close reading go hand-in-hand. I discovered that narrative medicine emerged in the early 2000s from the medicine and humanities movement that rose to prominence in the 1970s. Narrative medicine is thought of as the discipline of telling stories about illness — indeed, "honoring" the sick and suffering — from multiple perspectives, which culls its pedagogy from the fields of literary studies, film theory, philosophy, anthropology and social sciences. Narrative practice, on the other hand, encompasses various forms of training that aim to apply narrative ideas and skills to clinical conversations. Putting words on paper is an extension of narrative practice, one that aims to develop narrative practitioners rather than practitioners who have undertaken narrative studies.

I clearly aim to be both — a student of the narrative as well as a practitioner — as I travel on the road to discovery. It's a road that leads to the creation of meaning and understanding. It's a road to rejoicing and redeeming. It's a road that represents the coming together of cultures and genres in a place where everyone is welcome.

This is my pilgrimage. Join me.

NOTES AND SOURCES

WITH FEW EXCEPTIONS, all essays in this book were written between 2019 and 2023. They initially appeared online at one of several websites: KevinMD, MedPage Today, and Doximity. A few were first published in the *Physician Leadership Journal*, the *Journal of Medical Practice Management*, or the *Healthcare Administration Leadership & Management Journal*. The essays were edited and cross-referenced during the book's production. Medical references and citations to quotations were intentionally omitted in order to improve the continuity of reading. To access source information, readers can search each essay (by title) on the internet and click on hyperlinked text within the essay.

ALSO BY ARTHUR LAZARUS

*Neuroleptic Malignant Syndrome and
Related Conditions (co-author)*

Controversies in Managed Mental Health Care

Career Pathways in Psychiatry: Transition in Changing Times

*MD/MBA: Physicians on the New Frontier
of Medical Management*

www.ingramcontent.com/pod-product-compliance
Lightning Source LLC
Chambersburg PA
CBHW061137220326
41599CB00025B/4269